Joseph Smith
and
Herbal Medicine

A Brief Study of the Botanical Arts in Mormonism

Joseph Smith
and
Herbal Medicine

A Brief Study of the
Botanical Arts in
Mormonism

by

John Heinerman

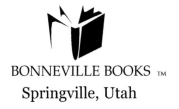

BONNEVILLE BOOKS ™
Springville, Utah

ISBN: 1-55517-505-8
v.2

Published by Bonneville Books
An imprint of Cedar Fort Inc.
925 N. Main, Springville, Utah 84663
Distributed by:

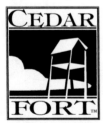

Typeset by Virginia Reeder
Cover design by Adam Ford
Cover design © 2000 by Adam Ford

Printed in the United States of America

TABLE OF CONTENTS

He causeth the grass to grow for the cattle, and for the
service of man . . .
(Psalms 104:14)

Introduction

Thursday, April 13, 1843 ...At 10 o'clock, the Emigrant and a great multitude of others assembled at the Temple and prayer by Elder Kimball. Joseph addressed the assembly and said:

"The doctors in this region don't know much.... DOCTORS WON'T TELL YOU HOW TO GO TO BE WELL. THEY WANT TO KILL OR CURE YOU TO GET YOUR MONEY.

Calomel doctors will give you calomel to cure a sliver in the big toe and not stop to know whether the stomach is empty or not. Calomel on an empty stomach will kill the patient and the lobelia doctors will do the same.

Point me out a patient and I will tell you whether calomel or lobelia will kill him or not...

If you feel any inconvenience, take some mild physic two or three times and then some bitters (herbs).

If you can't get anything else, take a little salt and cayenne pepper. If you can't get salt, take pecosia or gnaw down a butternut tree. Cut some boreset or horehound...

I will give you advice that will do you good. I bless you in the Name of Jesus Christ, Amen."

> (The Journals of Joseph Smith; under entry dated above; Church Historian's Office, Salt Lake City)

"...to get salvation we must not only do some things, but everything which God has commanded. Men may preach and practice everything except those things which God commands us to do, and will be damned at last. We may tithe mint and rue, and all manner of herbs, and still not obey the commandments of God. The object with me is to obey and teach others to obey God in just what He tells us to do. It mattereth not whether the principle is popular or unpopular, I WILL ALWAYS MAINTAIN A TRUE PRINCIPLE, even if I stand alone in it."

—The Prophet Joseph Smith

(Documentary History of The Church 6:223)

CHAPTER ONE

WITHOUT THE GIFT OF THE RESTORED GOSPEL

(The Smith Family and Doctors)

Joseph Smith, the Prophet of the Last Dispensation, was born in Vermont, the land of folk medicine as it is sometimes called. Coming from such a place rich in useful lore of the botanical sciences, it would be natural for his family to adopt many of the old home remedies for common cure in those primitive times. The healing with herbs and other natural substances seemed to have been the thing which was in vogue, considering the scarcity of doctors and limited knowledge of medical science in certain regions. Besides that, most country folk were too poor to afford anything else other than the simple advice prescribed by the local herbalist, or one skilled in the natural art of botany.

However, strange as this may seem, the Smiths, for some reason or another, came to rely upon physicians more than they did the botanic doctor. Of course, this can readily be understood why, when one considers the fact that they did not have the enlightenment of revelation to attend them, nor the graces, benefits and blessings of revealed scripture which would have shown them and made clear the proper manner in which to go when illness befell them. Only until after God, in His great and infinite Mercy, saw fit to shed forth Divine Light upon the children of men through a holy and inspired Seer, were they able to see the folly of their former ways, and repent themselves of such things, and adopt a wiser course more pleasing to the Lord, whom they earnestly sought in their daily prayers.

Several noted instances of sickness within their family demonstrates their faith and trust in the medical practitioner's arts over those of the herbalist. And, it is, perhaps, with these few incidents found in Joseph Smith's early youth, that the later opinion formed in regards to the medical profession which was entertained by him thereafter.

It was as a young lad that he suffered his first terrible and excruciating ordeal relative to the surgeon's knife. Mother Smith related the episode as follows:

> Joseph, our third son, having recovered from the typhus fever after something like two weeks' sickness, one day screamed out while sitting in a chair, with pain in his shoulder, and, in a very short time, he appeared to be in such agony that we feared the consequence would prove to be something very serious. We immediately sent for a doctor. When he arrived, and had examined the patient, he said that it was his opinion that this pain was occasioned by a sprain. But the child declared this could not be the case, as he had received no injury in any way whatsoever, but that a severe pain had seized him all at once, of the cause of which he was entirely ignorant.

> Notwithstanding the child's protestations, still the physician insisted that it must be a sprain, and consequently, he anointed his shoulder with some bone liniment; but this was of no advantage to him, for the pain continued the same after the anointing as before.

> When two weeks of extreme suffering had elapsed, the attendant physician concluded to make closer examination, whereupon he found that a large fever sore had gathered between his breast and shoulder. He immediately lanced it upon which it discharged fully a quart of purulent matter.

> As soon as the sore had discharged itself, the pain left it, and shot like lightning (using his own terms) down his side into the marrow of the bone of his leg, and soon became very severe. My poor boy, at this, was almost in despair, and he cried out, 'Oh, father! the pain is so severe, how can I bear it.'

> His leg soon began to swell, and he continued to suffer the greatest agony for the space of two weeks longer. During this time I carried him much of the time in my arms, in order to mitigate his suffering as much as possible, in consequence of which I was taken very ill myself. The anxiety of mind that I experienced, together with physical over-exertion, was too much for my constitution, and my nature sunk under it.

> Hyrum, who was rather remarkable for his tenderness and sympathy, now desired that he might take my place. As he was a good, trusty boy, we let him do so; and, in order to make the task as easy for him as possible, we laid Joseph upon a low bed, and Hyrum sat beside him, almost day and night, for some

4

considerable length of time, holding the affected part of his leg in his hands, and pressing it between them, so that his afflicted brother might be enabled to endure the pain, which was so excruciating that he was scarcely able to bear it.

At the end of three weeks we thought it advisable to send again for the surgeon. When he came, he made an incision of eight inches, on the front side of the leg, between the knee and ankle. This relieved the pain in a great measure, and the patient was quite comfortable until the wound began to heal, when the pain became as violent as ever.

The surgeon was called again, and he this time enlarged the wound, cutting the leg even to the bone. It commenced healing the second time, and as soon as it began to heal, it also began to swell again, which swelling continued to rise till we deemed it wisdom to call a council of surgeons; and when they met in consultation, they decided that amputation was the only remedy.

Soon after coming to this conclusion, they rode up to the door, and were invited into a room, apart from the one in which Joseph lay. They being seated, I addressed them thus:

'Gentlemen, what can you do to save my boy's leg?' They answered, 'We can do nothing; we have cut it open to the bone, and find it so affected that we consider the leg incurable, and that amputation is absolutely necessary in order to save his life.'

This was like a thunderbolt to me. I appealed to the principal surgeon, saying, 'Doctor Stone, can you not make another trial? Can you not, by cutting around the bone, take out the diseased part, and perhaps that which is sound will heal over, and by this means you will save his leg? You will not, you must not, take off his leg, until you try once more. I will not consent to let you enter his room until you make me this promise.'

After consulting a short time with each other, they agreed to do as I had requested, then went to see my suffering son. One of the doctors, on approaching his bed, said, 'My poor boy, we have come again.'

'Yes,' said Joseph, 'I see you have; but you have not come to take off my leg, have you, sir?' 'No,' replied the surgeon, 'it is your mother's request that we make one more effort, and that is

what we have now come for.'

...The surgeon commenced operating by boring into the bone of his leg, first on one side of the bone, where it was affected, then on the other side, after which they broke it off with a pair of forceps or pincers. They then took away the large pieces of the bone. When they broke off the first piece, Joseph screamed out so loudly that I could not forbear running to him. On my entering his room, he cried out, 'Oh, Mother, go back, go back; I do not want you to come in—I will try to tough it out, if you will go away.'

When the third piece was taken away, I burst into the room again—and oh, my God! what a spectacle for a mother's eyes. The wound torn open, the blood still gushing from it, and the bed literally covered with blood. Joseph was as pale as a corpse, and large drops of sweat were rolling down his face, whilst upon every feature was depicted the utmost agony.

I was immediately forced from the room, and detained until the operation was completed; but when the act was accomplished, Joseph put upon a clean bed, the room cleared of every appearance of blood, and the instruments which were used in the operation removed, I was permitted again to enter.

Joseph immediately commenced getting better, and from this time onward continued to mend until he became strong and healthy.[1]

After this trying circumstance, the boy, when a man, would always remember this agonizing event in his young life, and come to shun the surgeon's devices with a cold shudder of chilling memory.

His second experience had to do with prescribed medicine, and was without question, one of the main forces behind his determination to resist doctors thereafter, and seek for something better than the medical skills of men. It happened on this wise:

On the fifteenth day of November, 1825, about ten o'clock in the morning, Alvin was taken very sick with the bilious colic. He came to the house in much distress, and requested his father to go immediately for a physician. He accordingly went, and got one by the name of Greenwood, who, on arriving, immediately administered to the patient a heavy dose of calomel.[2] *I will here notice that this Doctor Greenwood was not*

6

the physician commonly employed by the family; he was brought in consequence of the family physician's absence. And on this account, as I suppose, Alvin at first refused to take the medicine, but by much persuasion he was prevailed on to do so.

This dose of calomel lodged in his stomach, and all the medicine which was freely administered by four very skilled physicians could not remove it.

On the third day of his sickness, Doctor McIntyre, whose services were usually employed by the family, as he was considered very skillful, was brought, and with him four other eminent physicians. But it was all in vain, their exertions proved unavailing, just as Alvin had said would be the case—he told them the calomel was still lodged in the same place, after some exertion had been made to carry it off, and that it must take his life.

On coming to this conclusion, he called Hyrum to him, and said, 'Hyrum, I must die...'

But when he came to Joseph, he said, 'I am now going to die, the distress which I suffer, and the feelings that I have, tell me my time is very short. I want you to be a good boy, and do everything that lies in your power to obtain the record. Be faithful in receiving instruction, and in keeping every commandment that is given you...'

...As I turned with the child to leave him, he said, 'Father, mother, brothers and sisters, farewell. I can now breathe out my life as calmly as a clock.' Saying this, he immediately closed his eyes in death.

Alvin was a youth of singular goodness of disposition— kind and amiable so that lamentations and mourning filled the whole neighborhood in which he resided.

By the request of the principal physician, Alvin was cut open, in order to discover, if it were possible, the cause of his death. On doing so, they found the calomel lodged in the upper bowels, untouched by anything which he had taken to remove it, and as near as possible in its natural state, surrounded as it was with gangrene.[3]

With the unfortunate loss of their beloved Alvin, through an overdosage of prescribed medicine, the family was at a loss for awhile, and had considerable cause to grieve at the death of so fine a young man.

Another experience which the family had had several years before this, also involved the use of medicine. In this instance, all of the medical doctor's prescribed drug did not alleviate the condition of the suffering soul; and, in the end, Mother Smith, of consequence, had to turn to the Lord to rescue her daughter from the throes of death.

The typhus fever came into Lebanon, and raged tremendously. Among the number seized with this complaint were, first, Sophronia; next Hyrum, who was taken while at school, and came home sick; then Alvin; in short, one after another was taken down, till all of the family, with the exception of myself and husband, were prostrated upon a bed of sickness.

Sophronia had a heavy siege. The physician attended upon her eighty-nine days, giving her medicine all the while; but on the ninetieth day, he said she was so far gone, it was not for her to receive any benefit from medicine, and for this cause he discontinued his attendance upon her. The ensuing night, she lay altogether motionless, with her eyes wide open, and with that peculiar aspect which bespeaks the near approach of death. As she thus lay, I gazed upon her as a mother looks upon the last shade of life in a darling child. In this moment of distraction, my husband and myself clasped our hands, fell upon our knees by the bedside, and poured out our grief to God, in prayer and supplication, beseeching Him to spare our child yet a little longer.

Did the Lord hear our petition? Yes, He most assuredly did, and before we rose to our feet, He gave us a testimony that she should recover. When he first arose from prayer, our child had, to all appearances, ceased breathing. I caught a blanket, threw it around her, then, taking her in my arms, commenced pacing the floor. Those present remonstrated against my doing as I did, saying, 'Mrs. Smith, it is all of no use; you are certainly crazy, your child is dead. Notwithstanding, I would not, for a moment, relinquish the hope of again seeing her breathe and live.

This recital, doubtless, will be uninteresting to some; but those who have experienced in life something of this kind are susceptible of feeling, and can sympathize with me. Are you a

8

mother who has been bereft of a child? Feel for your heart-strings, and then tell me how I felt with my expiring child pressed to my bosom! Would you at this trying moment feel to deny that God had 'power to save to the uttermost all who call on him?' I did not then; neither do I now.

At length she sobbed. I still pressed her to my breast, and continued to walk the floor. She sobbed again, then looked up into my face, and commenced breathing quite freely. My soul was satisfied, but my strength was gone. I laid my daughter on the bed, and sunk by her side, completely overpowered by the intensity of my feelings.

*From this time forward Sophronia continued mending, until she entirely recovered.*4

IN SUMMARY

1. Lacking divine wisdom, the Smiths were under the necessity of relying upon human resources, according to the best light they had in their possession then.

2. Young Joseph suffered tremendously under the able skill and profound learning of medical science in those times.

3. The best known medicine for that era, calomel, was directly responsible for the untimely death of Alvin Smith. An autopsy, requested by the physician who administered the lethal dose, proved conclusively that this had been the cause of his demise.

4. Prescribed medicine by skilled physicians, over an extended length of time, does not always help to alleviate the condition of sickness. Only faith and trust in God can guarantee a permanent deliverance, if it is meant to be so in the economy of Heaven.

CHAPTER TWO

THE DAWNING OF A NEW HORIZON
(A Short History of the Thomsonian Botanical Cure)

Sometime prior to the restoration of the Gospel in modern times, there was another evolution of intelligence which burst forth in all of its glory upon mankind everywhere. This was the age of botanical science, when it took its first great step forward in the form of a Samuel Thomson, America's original Botanic Physician. For, with him rests the credit and glory of having founded and established a system of herbology which became the standard of healing for many sound-thinking people in those days.

In his later manhood, when the Prophet Joseph Smith became aware of such a wonderful system of cure, he had these fine commendations to offer about it:

Joseph Smith said that Thomson was as much inspired to bring forth his principle of practice according to the dignity and importance of it as he was to introduce the Gospel.[1]

In other words, the Prophet was equating the Gentile Thomson on the same level with himself, saying as it were that BOTH HAD BEEN INSPIRED OF GOD in their respective sciences—he, Joseph, in his new-found theology; and Mr. Thomson in his herbal medicine.

Another testimonial offered as proof of both men's divine calling is this:

Then we should look on those principles (Thomson Botanical Cure) as an appendix to the Gospel as a temporal salvation. It was introduced nearly contemporary with the Gospel and in its main features runs in sympathy with the Gospel, even the 'Word of Wisdom' and Thomsonian run together and strengthen each other instead of coming in collision with each other.

Thomson was educated the same as Joseph Smith was; he had not much experience the same as Joseph Smith and was not of high parentage so thought by the world the same as Joseph Smith was. They tried to kill him the same as Joseph Smith; they lanced him the same as they did Joseph Smith and did everything in their power to stop its progress, but could not do it because it was of inspiration and, of course, of divine origin like Joseph Smith, 'a mission,' and has never lacked opposition ever since it was introduced, just like Mormonism; and that is one evidence of its being correct, for the Prophets have said there must needs be an opposition in all things, and they have also said it must needs be that offenses come, but woe unto them by whom they come.[2]

Priddy Meeks, an early Mormon pioneer, and himself a botanic physician after the Thomsonian manner, declared that "the Lord was in the whole affair" of him entering herbal medicine. Of this background he provides the following:

I stopped on the Illinois River five of six miles above Meridocia, a town on the river, a sicklier place I never want to see. Here I bought me a nice little farm, and established a wood yard. Here I lost Huldah with the whooping cough; or in other words she was killed by the doctors, whom I was opposed to having anything to do with her, only the folks over-persuaded me, and I am convinced that his medicine killed her.

Here when the sickly season of the year came on, I visited many of the sick, and was very successful in relieving them with roots and herbs. So much so that the community insisted I should quit work and go to doctoring. Such an idea had never entered my mind. I said to them that I knew nothing about doctoring; they said, 'You beat all the doctors.'

That expression brought me to my studies and I saw that it was a fact, and I could not deny it. I studied much to know what was my duty to God and to mankind and myself and family. I saw my weakness and want of education, being raised in the backwoods with my gun on my shoulder, having no correspondence with the bulk of the community and knew nothing of the ways of the world. Here was a trial you may be sure, for me to come in contact with learned doctors; I would not know what to say and would appear as a dunce.

About this time I had a letter from my brother-in-law, stating that he had important business and wanted to see me, and I must come immediately. He lived about a hundred miles off in Macon County, Illinois. I went and left my sick wife, who had been sick for two years. Her case was so complicated that I did not know what to do; neither did the doctors, that had exhausted their skill without benefit, know what to do next.

When I saw my brother-in-law, whose name was Priddy Nahurin, he said that he only wanted a visit of me, that was all; but the Lord was in the whole affair, for I met a man there by the name of James Miller, whom I previously knew in Kentucky. He had gotten to be a Thomsonian doctor. He told me I could cure my wife myself if I had Thomson's 'New Guide to Health.'

I traveled thirty miles with him a-going home. I learned more from him that day than I ever knew before about doctoring. Arriving at home, I told my wife of the interview I had with Miller, and was a-going to buy the books that he recommended. She replied, 'You had better keep the money to raise the children with; for if the skill that has been exhausted by experienced doctors could not cure me, it is not reasonable to think that you could do any better.' But I could not rest satisfied until I got the books; and just two weeks to the day from the day I got the books, I put out into the woods to collect the medicine and by following the directions of the books, I made a sound woman of her. This gave such an impetus to the anxiety of the people about my success that it seemed like going against wind and tide to withstand their influence, for me to go into doctoring. And from that time henceforth my labors began with the sick.[3]

To give the reader somewhat of an insight into the Thomsonian method of herbal cure, and the inspired man who conceived it, the following is extended for the reader's kind perusal:

Samuel Thomson, the original botanic physician, was born February 9, 1769, at Alstead, New Hampshire. Though entirely self-taught, according to his own narrative, his biographer, a 'regular' physician, declares Thomson was a remarkable man with an extraordinary career.[4]

The summer he was four and a half years of age, Thomson says he herded geese and hunted cows. Emulating these natural foragers one day young Thomson ate a generous helping of lobelia pods. The plant is a natural emetic[5], and the result 'was so remarkable I never forgot it!' He later perpetrated jokes on his playmates, inducing them to eat lobelia pods, and experience the effects. With a natural leaning toward the healing profession, Thomson, through years of observation and study, gleaned all the information available on the healing properties of plants, and gathered from the older men and women many useful facts for the treatment of illness. While yet a youth, he gained quite a reputation for healing disease; and his own special curative system was developed and perfected by practice in his own family circle and neighborhood.

Lobelia, the 'Emetic Herb,' never failed him, he says, and became the cornerstone of his healing system, plus enemas, plus cayenne pepper (heat) and hot sweat baths. All these agents were obviously unusual yet very needful in those long inactive New Hampshire winters. From his ministrations, hosts of patients came to regard him as a gifted genius. Health circles and botanic societies took the place of neighborhood quilting bees and young Thomson regularly rode the circuit of sick homes in New England.

Presented in an age and to a people unacquainted with the commoner causes and consequences of discomfort, distress and disease, Thomson's cayenne pepper stimulated the system while his emetic and purge produced a cleanliness akin to godliness; also the enema made many fast friends, while the innovation of the steam or sweat bath allayed the people's fevers, quieted their nerves, and made for peaceful sickrooms, and often stayed the hand of death.

Thomson missed being fitted into the substructure of the medical profession by ungenerously securing a patent on his discovery of the actions of Lobelia, if he did not in fact impugn far too much intelligence and power to his babyhood emetic. Then he made things worse by trying to explain what he did not understand. His idea was that heat is a manifestation of life and that cold is the cause of disease. 'All disorders arise directly from obstructed perspiration, which is always caused by cold, or want of heat,' he explained. Boiled down, the Thomsonian System was: 1. Cleanse the body with lobelia (emetic) and enemas; 2. Restore the lost heat by cayenne pepper inside; hot pads and especially steam or vapor cabinet baths externally; 3. Finally, carry away the residue of 'canker' by doses of bayberry, sumac, red raspberry and so forth.

But, for his self-acquired erudition he was given the 'raspberry,' by most other practitioners, including many of his own student healers. They objected to his claims of proprietorship and to his copyrighted explanation. Once in 1809, he was indicted for murder for a case that did not yield; and the finger of ridicule was pointed at him by those who did not sympathize and believe with him. Thus while he opened his first office in Beverly, Massachusetts, he shortly moved to Boston—where he maintained headquarters through the rest of his career.

Thomson's first patent was issued by the U.S. Government on March 3, 1813, after a great deal of vexations and delay. Armed with this significant document, with a religious faith in his curative system, and with a vindictive hate for the regular medical profession, he went forth to slay the demon disease, in all its forms. Through newspaper, advertisements, and handbills he told the world of his invincible system, and by the powers of oratory derided the prevalent medical methods of bleeding their patients twice a day through ten-day courses, for fevers, and for loading already clogged human bodies with mercury and opium. The Captains in his crusading army were accorded the right to use the system and to sell the rights to others, which right in all cases was to cost $20, and to be granted only by the hand of Thomson—who doubtless in this way split commissions on the resales. The lieutenants in Thomson's army had only the right to heal, Thomsonian method, for their $20; but the privates were the public at large, and all had a right to be healed.

The fad swept the country like wildfire; and the organized opposition of the 'regular' Medicos only helped to spread the new doctrine, like whipping a fire among the leaves, as he said. Each edition of the instruction leaflet was larger than its predecessor—until in 1822 it appeared in book form, truly a compendium of health! Then a difficulty with his printer led to another schism, and with it plagiarizing pirates published the essence of his work and offered it for three bits apiece. The fire in the leaves had become a forest fire. Again this backfire was kindled by a new government patent, issued January 23, 1823, covering 'the use of steam to produce perspiration.' To make matters worse, Thomson's army was not organized, were widely scattered, and weren't working at it all the time. In short, they lacked tangible, effective leadership, and left Thomson fighting the windmills of the country, almost single-handedly. From 1826 to 1836 he had 'been six times in and through the State of Ohio' whence the Thomsonian System had spread faster than the older schools of healing.

Botanic societies, health circles, eclectic[6] and botanic physicians were springing up throughout the East, which knew not Thomson! Dr. Wooster Beach in 1827 founded an Infirmary in New York, out of which grew the Reformed Medical College—the inception of the Eclectic[6] System—opposed to the blood-letting M.D.'s—and to the monopolistic unethical Thomsonians alike—yet it adopted many of the medicines amid principles of the former, and adhered to the cardinal teachings of Thomson. The Reformed Medical College established a branch school at Worthington, Ohio, in 1832, which threatened to steal Thomson's thunder down to a whisper.

Independently of all medical factions, came Constantine S. Rafinesque with 'The Medical Flora of the United States' published in Philadelphia in 1828. Rafinesque had traveled extensively over the Mississippi Valley, then populated partly with the Native Indians, from whom he obtained much useful information. His unique work thus became another textbook for the botanics and the eclectics alike.

Parenthetically, Thomson may have had some enterprising Indian neighbors in his formative days—Josiah Gregg, Commerce of the Prairies, 1831-39, published 1844, Vol. 2, pp. 296–7, says the Indians of the Prairies had 'become acquainted with the medical virtues of many of their indigenous plants, which are often used in connection with the vapor sweat, and cold bath; wherefore we may consider them as the primitive Thomsonians.'

Dr. Alva Curtis, loyal Thomsonian, opened a 'Physico—Medical College of Ohio' in Cincinnati in 1836. As an advocate of a new system, Dr. Curtis was 'host' in himself, but as a torch-carrying school teacher, he flickered out in a few years. There—upon the Worthington, Ohio, Reformed Medical College moved to Cincinnati in 1845 and became the Eclectic Medical Institute. Thus, says Dr. J. M. Ball, Medical Historian, 'The Botanic, Eclectic and Physio-Medical sects...can be traced to Thomson.'

The strictly botanical schools gradually petered out; they changed their names and modified their methods. The botanic courses persisted, however, especially in the Ohio hotbed of Thomsonianism, for a great many years; and the Thomsonian principles were handed down traditionally even to the present generation. There are still plenty of reputable physicians recommending colonics and cabinet baths; and the aroma of sassafras tea in the city restaurants and the country homes of the land today as a tonic and blood tuner-up in a fragrance tracting all the way back to Doctor Thomson, a full century ago!

That 'steam doctor' Thomson was a benefactor among the Mormons, as among other groups, there is no doubt. 'Glory enough for one man,' it was said of him! He 'saved more millions of human beings from a miserable life and a premature grave than the whole United States contained in the days of Washington, by a system which spread more rapidly than any other system ever did upon its own merits!'

Dr. Thomson died October 4, 1843, in Boston, aged 75 years—a remarkable span for a man in those days!

John Thomson, a son, carried on actively for many years, but contributed nothing to his father's well-developed three-leg healing system—of purging, heating, and sweating; except his own picture replaced the father's on the diplomas! Son John still (in 1852) sold, for $6.00, the twenty dollar 'copyright of preparing and using the system of medical practice secured to Samuel Thomson by letters of patent, and (the purchaser) is thus constituted a member of the Thomsonian Friendly Botanic Society and is entitled to participate in its privileges. Whatever those privileges were!

Miss Blanche E. Rose in her thesis, 'The History of Medicine in Utah'—gives a typewritten copy of the Thomsonian Certificate issued to Dr. Willard Richards as a sub-agent, at Richmond, Massachusetts, by Joseph Skims, 'agent' for S. Thomson, October 3, 1833. Richards was then 29 years of age. Realizing he had only a diploma and no training, he moved to Boston and entered the Thomsonian Infirmary. He practiced for some time under Dr. Samuel Thomson himself. In 1835 he moved to Holliston, Massachusetts, and continued the practice of his profession. There he turned to Mormonism, through his cousin Brigham Young.

But the Thomsonian diploma authorized and empowered Richards to 'administer, use and sell the medicine secured to Samuel Thomson by letters patent,' and 'also to sell family rights (signed by Skims) with a copy of Thomson's 'New Guide to Health, and a narrative of his life,' for twenty dollars.

Miss Rose also gives the following supplement to the Thomsonian certificate: entitled 'Extra and Confidential to Agents' (to be given at discretion to the purchaser of rights). To prepare, add 4 lbs. white sugar, pound into a paste 2 oz. poplar bark, 2 oz. bayberry, 2 oz. golden seal, 2 oz. cloves, 2 oz,.cinnamon, 2 oz. nerve powder, 1 oz. cayenne, 1/2 bitter roots. Mix and knead with pestle in mortar until it becomes a thick dough. Add 1 tip penny-royal. Pound well together and roll in a loaf or make pills.

'For all diseases caused by colds and other diseases without regard to names:

'The above powder with the same weight of sugar, will make good spice bitters for wine. Put 2 oz. of the compound into one quart.

'Powders may be eaten dry, or taken in hot water with more sugar. No spirit is recommended in the medicine.

'Notice to Agent:

'Do justice to yourself and proprietor and public. Sell no rights to doctors or those who have studied their authors for a rule of practice, as they will most assuredly corrupt the system, as some have already done.'

'KEEP NO POISONOUS DRUGS IN YOUR SHOP,' as no one should sell to others what he would not use himself; or suffer any human blood to be shed, with the lancet or otherwise, by your consent.[7]

IN SUMMARY

1. The Prophet Joseph Smith said that Mr. Thomson, the botanic physician, was just as inspired in his profession, as what he (Joseph) had been in his.

2. From this declaration of the Prophet's, we can then safely assume that HERBAL MEDICINE (as first introduced by Mr. Thomson through his system) is AS MUCH A DIVINELY INSPIRED PRINCIPLE FROM HEAVEN AS THE GOSPEL IS!

3. Priddy Meeks said that Mr. Thomson's Botanical Cure was AN ADDITION TO THE GOSPEL, and PART OF OUR TEMPORAL SALVA-TION! Complementing the Word of Wisdom very nicely, Thomson's HERBAL MEDICINE WAS PART OF THE GOSPEL OF JESUS CHRIST!

4. The origin of Thomson's Botanical Cure and Joseph Smith's Restored Gospel paralleled each other significantly in their origin. Both systems of science had been born in much persecution and hardship.

5. The backgrounds of both men were quite similar. Both were from the New England States; both had experienced unpleasant episodes with medical physicians in their life; and both were persecuted for the truth they believed in and so strongly advocated.

6. Both Mr. Thomson and Priddy Meeks despised medical doctors with a passion!

7. The Thomsonian System, as it became developed, met with intense opposition from the known Medical Association then.

8. The Thomsonian System became somewhat exploited, both by Mr. Thomson himself as well as others. Originally conceived as a benefit for people, it became somewhat of a business speculation later on through the crass commercialism of its day. Despite these capitalistic opportunities, which it gained, it did not lose any of its apparent healing effectiveness with the people in general.

9. Those who were agents for the Thomsonian System were not allowed to carry, sell, or dispense any kind of medical drugs whatsoever. This meant that DR. WILLARD RICHARDS WAS AN HERBAL DOCTOR AND NOT A MEDICAL PRACTITIONER, as some believe him to have been in history.

CHAPTER THREE

BENEATH THE SPLENDID RAYS OF TRUTH

(Joseph Smith and Herbal Medicine)

Apparently, the first real intimation the Prophet Joseph Smith had of herbal medicine and the fact that it was Divinely-approved, came about while he was engaged in the translation of that sacred record, the Golden Plates received from Moroni, into the present form of the Book of Mormon. As he was thus endeavoring to pursue his inspired labors in this direction, he read the following sacred words from that precious and holy work:

> And there were some who died with fevers, but which at some seasons of the year was very frequent in the land; but not so much so with fevers, because of the excellent qualities of the many plants and roots which God prepared to remove the cause of diseases, to which men were subject by the nature of the climate.[1]

Here it was, plain as day; God speaking to modern man once again, and setting down as clear as crystal the manner in which he ought to heal himself.

As he read these words of wisdom, he must have reflected back upon the unpleasant associations he and his family had had with medical men in the past. Or, as one writer so graphically portrayed it:

> Alvin's death alone was enough to sadden Joseph. But certain associations surrounding it may have made Joseph's grief still more bitter. Alvin had died, it seemed to Joseph, because the family had relied on doctors and their medicines. Certainly he could never have forgotten the sight of those pills. Later his preaching against calomel was so effective that its influence was felt for years.[2]

Thus, it seems that a combination of both the scripture from holy writ and a vivid recollection of a bitter past, served to incline his mind toward herbal medicine for sure, and away from medical science.

His mind became further influenced by Heavenly things in this direction, when the Lord revealed to him, in a revelation given February 9, 1831, the precise and exact manner in which the Saints of the Most High were to be treated and dealt with in accordance to the laws of nature, when sickness, disease, and pain prevailed among them.

And whosoever among you are sick, and have not faith
to be healed, but believe, shall be nourished with all tenderness,
with herbs and mild food, and that not by the hand of an enemy.[3]

Now it is interesting to note that when the Lord gave this commandment to man, He singled out those who were to receive the benefits and blessings of herbal medicine and those who were not to. He mentions that those "among you" who "are sick" and have not faith to be healed, but "believe," were to be THE ONLY ONES unto whom such things as what He had just prescribed, were to be administered. In other words, He was clearly saying that the application of herbs and mild food were to be given just to those who believed in these things, though they had no faith in which to be healed, AND NOT TO THE UNBELIEVER! Thus, God established a precedent then, which if in modern times was followed, would result in less persecution upon them who trust and confide in such remedies and solutions. In a word, He was saying: let those who believe in herbs, use herbs; and let those who do not believe in herbs, not use them.

Here is the beautiful principle of free agency incorporated with Heavenly wisdom; how Divine; how majestic! and how remarkable are the ways of the Lord when followed. By official commandment, it is not for those who believe in herbs and use them, to make an attempt drowning others in their teas and liquids. Nor, is it for those who look to the men in white for their medical salvation, to remark disparagingly and abuse those humble followers engaged in such "strange" practices and "weird" beliefs. Each to his own, and to have contentment between them both. Such are the ways of righteousness, with everything in good and proper order, and everyone to his or her own lifestyle of choosing. For, of such, are the ways of the Lord.

And again the Lord spoke, by way of commandment, as to the proper course which should be taken in all things, when He delivered this message in a revelation given February 27, 1833:

And again, verily I say unto you, all wholesome herbs God hath ordained for the constitution, nature, and use of man—

Every herb in the season thereof, and every fruit in the season thereof; all these to be used with prudence and thanks-giving.[4]

This Word of Wisdom, given as an admonishment and later adopted as a law into the Church, is interesting by way of several factors:

First, the principle definition of what an "herb" precisely is—

A plant of economic value; specifically, one used for MEDICINAL PURPOSES, *or for its sweet scent or flavor.*[5]

Second, the chief interpretation of the word "fruit" in a botanical sense of science.

Botany. (a) In general, any product of fertilization with its modified envelopes or appendages...(I,) *specifically,* and more commonly, the ripened ovary of a seed plant and its contents, including such adjacent tissues as may be inseparably connected with it, as the pod of a pea, the capsule of many annuals, etc. Fruits are *simple,* the product of a single enlarged ovary; *aggregate,* the product of the several ovaries of a single flower; or *collective* (multiple), derived from the more or less fused ovaries of several flowers. The *principal kinds of fruit* (in the botanical sense) are:

SIMPLE

legume (pad): bean, pea, Caryopsis (grain): wheat, Indian corn.

Berry: grape, tomato.
Drupe (stone fruit): plum, olive.
Rome: apple, pear.
AGGREGATE
Strawberry, raspberry, magnolia.
COLLECTIVE (MULTIPLE)
Mulberry, fig, pineapple. [6]

Now, the above facts were not meant to be given as a short dissertation in the science of botany, but to help clarify a misunderstanding many Latter-day Saints have in regards to the Word of Wisdom. It is commonly thought to be the case that when God meant the "herb," He was referring to just vegetables alone; and when He meant the "fruit," he was referring to items like peaches, pears, apples, and other assorted like things which only grow on trees. But THIS is NOT THE CASE AND HAS NEVER BEEN, EITHER.

To be specific about the matter: when He gave the Word of Wisdom, he was, first of all, referring to the fact that He had ordained and given the herbs of the field to be for the use and benefit of man. Or, to be more pronounced about the matter in discussion: HE HAD ALLOWED FOR CERTAIN PLANTS TO BE USED AS MEDICINE IN THE CONSTITUTION AND NATURE OF MAN! He never said one word about the drugs obtained through chemical science. He was speaking in a botanical sense when He gave that commandment to the Church, to be observed by all, if they so chose to do.

If this is rather staggering for the reader to conceive of, then kindly go back and re-read the first verse of the quoted scripture previously given on the opposite page. And you will find that God specifically refers to herbs in one sentence, and to fruits in another. Two different things, in two different verses altogether. The dictionary consulted is quite reputable and the definition furnished very explicit in this matter, and is certainly conclusive evidence that AN HERB IS A PLANT USED FOR MEDICINAL PURPOSES, or for the seasoning of food.

Secondly, the "fruit" referred to by Him, in the second verse of that revelation, is with regards to VEGETABLES as well as the ordinary tree-grown kind, harvested in the usual manner of picking. Even wheat of the grain family is considered "fruit" under the botanical sense of classification.

In regards to the Word of Wisdom and how closely it is connected with herbal medicine, a prominent Latter-day Saint botanic physician, Priddy Meeks, had this injunction to give the Mormon people:

> One main object I have in view is to turn the hearts of the Saints to the Word of Wisdom that the wisdom may be sanctified in the hearts of the Saints, to the exclusion of the popular physicians and their poison medicine of the present day, and simplify every one among the Saints to one name for each article, with one meaning to that name; that children may not err thereby,

ignoring all the customs and fashions and technicalities of the dead languages that have caused the death of thousands of our dear friends, and obey the word of the Lord by using these herbs that He says He has ordained for the 'Constitution,' 'Nature,' and 'Use of Man.'

Also to simplify the practice of midwifery down to its natural wants: 'And what are its natural wants?' Nothing but to have the obstructions removed, and you cannot prevent delivery only at the expense of life because it's the law of nature which is the law of life, which is the law of God, which is immutable. (Did you ever know a squaw to die in childbirth?)

Then away with your pretended science of midwifery. There is more harm done by it than good.

When the pain flats out and stops, just remove the obstructions and the pains will return, and come as a natural consequence being a natural call the same as any other call of nature. Precisely there is no difference in the principle, and the Lord has ordained means among those anti-poison herbs adapted to that very purpose.

When the foregoing conditions are reached, we then can raise all the medicines needful in our gardens which are well adapted to human culture, but as yet cannot furnish them all on account of climatic difference. Then will be the time when there is no danger of poisoning our families and bringing them to a premature grave. We then shall be delivered from THE GREATEST CURSE THAT EVER VISITED THE HUMAN FAMILY *since Adam first set his foot on this earth. May God help to speed on the time when the Saints may enjoy the blessings of such times and Israel gathered and Zion built up and Him on the throne whose right it is to reign. When the foregoing condition takes place among the community there will be no more schools of midwifery.*[7]

What the author is attempting to do here is not to discredit medical science, or to push herbal remedies, but to set down in clear, definable language the distinct advice of God, which is so clear and concise upon the subject, that even a child possessed of mediocre intelligence, could readily grasp the same, once it had been all explained to his satisfaction and good. In other words, in the Word of Wisdom was given the formula by which all men could live right, if followed and applied;

both for their physical appetites as well as for their good being of health. He provided a way in which man might eat right and a logical manner in which he may be cured right, also. If strictly adhered to, and obeyed in the explicit sense that it was given, a lot of the professional services available today for man's nutrition and health would be done away with, and have no place in our society whatsoever. But then and again, man is his own agent and may dictate for himself the affairs of his wants and the rejections of his wishes. This is his prerogative and privilege and he may live accordingly; and also pay accordingly, for those things which he adopts that are *contrary* to the laws of Heaven, to which a most severe penalty for disobedience has been attached.

Through His latter-day Seer and Revelator the Lord confirmed this fact, when He had his holy prophet declare:

There is a law, irrevocably decreed in heaven before the foundations of this world, upon which all blessings are predicated—

And when we obtain any blessing from God, it is by obedience to that law upon which it is.

Joseph Smith sought to do this, and remembering what his brother Alvin had told him to do in obeying the commandments of the Lord, he endeavored to practice sound principles of good eating habits and allow himself to be nursed and doctored by those skilled in the arts of herbal medicine. As a result, he enjoyed fine physical health, generally speaking (save for an occasion or two, when he was severely poisoned by an enemy) and was pretty-much free from sickness and illness (except occasional fatigue and exhaustion due to the strenuous work-load which rested upon his shoulders to perform).

As a matter of fact, his whole family became adapted to this heavenly method of cure, after the Lord gave certain, specific revelations on the matter to their son and brother. We find the Prophet recording upon one such an occasion, when his father was severely ill:

Went to visit my father. Found him very low. Administered some mild herbs to the commandment. May God grant to restore him immediately to health for Christ the Redeemer's sake, Amen.[9]

The reader's attention will kindly be called again to the statement of he "administered some mild herbs AGREEABLE TO THE COMMANDMENT!" He was only doing that thing which God had instructed him to do. Had it not been for this, he would have followed in the usual footsteps of his father and mother, and forthwith, summoned a medical physician immediately, which seems to have been the tradition in the Smith household for a long time, until the light of the Lord touched the young man's mind and memory with better things than what they had known.

Now, apparently the instructions he followed in the commandment of the Word of Wisdom, did not serve enough to help his father, and he found him "failing very fast" and "very sick." So, what did he do? Did he lose faith in God and send for a medical doctor immediately? Did he believe that "faith without works is dead," and feel to submit his faith into the hands of licensed practitioners? No, HE DID NOT! He submitted himself and his faith into the hands of the living God, and performed the following ordinance of life upon his dear father, as given in his own authoritative words:

> In secret prayer in the morning, the Lord said, 'My Servant, thy Father shall live. 'I waited on him all this day with my heart raised to God in the Name of Jesus Christ that he would restore him to health again, that I might be blessed with his company and advice, esteeming it one of the greatest earthly blessings to be blessed with the society of parents, whose mature years and experience renders them capable of administering the most wholesome advice. At evening Bro. David Whitmer came in. We called on the Lord in mighty prayer in the Name of Jesus Christ and laid our hands on him, and rebuked the disease and God heard and answered our prayers to the great joy and satisfaction of our souls. Our aged Father arose and dressed himself, shouted and praised the Lord; called Bro. Wm. Smith, who had retired to rest that he might praise the Lord with us by joining in songs of praise to the Most High...[10]

He had found that herbs, like regularly prescribed medicine from a doctor, can also fail at times, too. This instance with his beloved father, and the unhappy episode of calomel with his dear brother, Alvin, had taught him that neither can be very sure at times; and when so, then the next best thing to do, was to turn to God, and put full and complete trust in Him. Or, as he would say, "agreeable to commandment":

> And the elders of the church, two or more, shall be called, and shall pray for and lay their hands upon them in my name; and if they die they shall die unto me, and if they live they shall live unto me.[11]

Which is what he did in this case, after the standard procedures employed with the herbs had been followed; and his father was healed immediately.

But the Prophet's over-all confidence in herbal medicine was such that he undertook to surround himself with the very best botanic physicians available for those times.

> *Thus, many of the doctors of early Mormondom, but not all, were Thomsonians. At least three Thomsonians reached high positions in the Church. One was Frederick G. Williams; the other two were the Richards' brothers, Levi and Willard. In their positions they exerted considerable influence on the attitude of the Church toward medicine. Dr. Williams was Joseph Smith's counselor during the early formative period of the church, Levi was Joseph Smith's personal physician toward the end of his life, and Willard became first counselor to his cousin, Brigham Young, and the editor of the Church organ, the Deseret News. Thus, the seeds of the antipathy between Thomsonian or lobelia doctors and orthodox or 'poison' doctors, as the Utah pioneers called them, were sown in the minds of Church members.[12]*

The Prophet's personal attitude and views toward these men, may also be seen in the following:

> *When, in 1837, Willard Richards, a convert to the Church from Massachusetts, came to Kirtland, Ohio (then Joseph's headquarters), he arrived as a 'botanic physician.' He treated his patients with 'warm medicines,' of which cayenne and lobelia were two principal ingredients. He also used mild herbs, but no 'poison pills.' Richards had learned his method from its originator, Samuel Thomson, in Massachusetts. Considerable illness in Richard's parent's family had led him to take Thomson's six-week course in Boston, and he later underwent a thorough apprenticeship. (The course at the College of Medicine in Pittsfield, Massachusetts—comparable at that time to Harvard in enrollment—was only a fourteen-week term.[13]*

> *Willard's brother, Levi, also joined the Church as a physician. But while Levi was in England on a mission, Willard wrote him to bring home a set of watchmaker's tools; he did not think Levi could earn much in Nauvoo through medicine. Joseph, said Willard, was dead set against the practice of medicine.*

> But while Levi was traveling back to Nauvoo, Willard's wife, Jeannetta, became ill. Levi was in St. Louis waiting for the frozen Mississippi's ice to break up so he could continue his trip when Willard—with Jeannetta's approval—wrote for his professional advice.

> The time came when Joseph Smith himself called upon Levi to attend him, and he once declared there was no better doctor in the world. But Levi prescribed no calomel.

But an even better glimpse into how Joseph Smith rated these men in comparison to the standard medical skills available in those days, is provided with this:

> Levi...was a surgeon-general of the Nauvoo Legion, and physician to the Prophet Joseph Smith and his brother Hyrum. In the Prophet's journal under the date of April 19, 1843, is found this entry. 'I will say that that man (Levi Richards) is the best physician I have ever been acquainted with .[15]

Joseph Smith was no fool! He knew which procedure to follow, and what type of men to have around him. When his father was sick, he tried the one and then the other. If the administration would have failed, then he would have quietly resigned himself to the fact that his father must die, and delivered the old man up to God in peace without any further struggle. For, he knew too well by heart the scripture which he had translated in the Book of Mormon:

> CURSED is he that putteth his trust in the arm of flesh. Yea, CURSED is he that putteth his trust in man, or maketh flesh his arm.[16]

He was not about to risk his life nor his father's life by submitting to the services of medical men, and thereby, possibly incurring the wrath and indignation of an angry and displeased God. No, he was much too intelligent for that terrible consequence to have befallen him, and hence, felt to declare within his soul, as the Prophet did anciently:

> O Lord, I have trusted in thee, and I will trust in thee forever. l will not put my trust in the arm of flesh. [17]

Jesus said, "If ye love me, keep my commandments."[18] Joseph Smith had seen the man who had spoken those words. He had heard His Voice and beheld His Glory. And, he simply could not disobey the Man who had given him the commandment of the Word of Wisdom.

The Word of Wisdom, as the Lord had declared it to him, made specific mention of the use of herbs for "the constitution and nature of man." And he knew what the Lord expected of him, as His Servant and leader of His People. He must set the precedent for everyone else to follow, in order that all might be saved. Only once before, in his early manhood, had he disobeyed the Lord and gave into the hands of a wicked man, one hundred sixteen pages of the written manuscript of the Book of Mormon. These had been lost; and for this act of disobedience, God chastized him sorely and withdrew His Spirit for the approximate space of six months, until He felt His young servant had sufficiently paid the penalty for his unintentional mistake.

From this swift and vivid lesson, Joseph Smith had keenly learned that when God commands, MAN MUST OBEY, or suffer for his transgressions. Because he loved the Lord, he kept the commandment of the Word of Wisdom, and employed only herbal remedies and herbal doctors whenever sickness was found in his midst. If we love the Lord, and revere the sacred and honorable name of Joseph Smith so highly today, ought we not to be doing the same also, and keep them as he kept them?

IN SUMMARY

1. Joseph Smith believed that the death of his dear brother, Alvin, had been partly caused by the family's reliance on medical doctors and their medicine. "Certainly he could never have forgotten the sight of those pills."

2. The Book of Mormon effectively points out that the ancient Nephites who inhabited this continent a long time ago, used herbs and roots to nurse their sick back to health.

3. Modern revelation, as found in the Doctrine and Covenants, tells us to do the very same thing, also, with the inclusion of mild food, appended therewith.

4. A careful examination of the Word of Wisdom, and proper definition of the words "herb" and "fruit" clearly show that God had reference to herbal medicine as a means of healing.

5. Just because the Word of Wisdom states that herbs are to be

used for "the constitution, nature and use of man," it does not mean that everybody is to rely upon herbal medicine as their only medium of health. But, that such things are to be given only to them that "believe" in them. A man's free agency must not be imposed upon, neither his rights of choosing infringed upon. God has made this aspect perfectly clear.

6. When we keep a law, we receive a blessing. The Word of Wisdom, as we now understand it, is a direct law from God, obedience to it, in the *precise* language which it is given, will yield a blessing of health to those who submit themselves to it. For those who choose to adopt another plan and method of action, will be denied this blessing. It's as simple as that!

7. Joseph Smith administered herbs to his sick father, in accordance with the commandment given him previously. This shows that he obeyed the Word of Wisdom in its plainest and simplest terms; and took it literally to mean just what it said.

8. Though he was faithful in this respect and true to the Word of God, it did not produce for him, the gratifying results he had hoped it would have.

9. By following the next commandment of God then, and turning to administration, he healed his sick father of his destitute condition and God made the old man well again.

10. Joseph Smith *always* surrounded himself with botanic physicians who believed in the herbal ways of healing.

11. Such men had considerable influence upon the Church in his time, because of their standing with him.

12. Joseph Smith was dead set against the practice of medicine; and declared that his own personal herbalist, Levi Richards, was the BEST PHYSICIAN he'd ever known.

13. Joseph Smith believed in herbalism because he loved the Lord and knew that that was what God wanted of him. If we love the Lord, should we not do the same likewise?

CHAPTER FOUR

"COME FOLLOW ME"

(The Use and Practice of Herbal Medicine in Nauvoo)

'Come, follow me,' the Saviour said;
Then let us in His footsteps tread.
For thus alone can we be one
With God's own loved, begotten Son.

Come, follow me—a simple phrase,
Yet truth's sublime, effulgent rays
Are in these simple words combined
To urge, inspire the human mind.

Is it enough alone to know
That we must follow Him below,
While trav'ling thro' this vale of tears?
No, this extends to holier spheres.

Not only shall we emulate
His course while in this earthly state,
But when we're freed from present cares,
If, with our Lord we would be heirs.

We must the onward path pursue
As wider fields expand to view,
And follow Him unceasingly
Whate' er our lot or sphere may be.[1]

The Saints of Nauvoo believed that inasmuch as their Prophet was following the injunctions of the Savior, and obeying His principles, they ought to do the same. As early as Far West, Missouri, the services of one of the leading botanical physicians in the Church was called upon:

> *I, Levi Richards, a resident of Quincy, Adams County,*
> *Illinois, practitioner of medicine, certify that in the year one*
> *thousand eight hundred and thirty-eight, I was a citizen of Far*
> *West, Caldwell County, Missouri, and that in the fall of said year,*

I saw the city invaded by a numerous soldiery...

I was called to extract lead, dress the wounds, etc., for several persons (Saints) who were shot in the above siege, two of of whom died.[2]

Of course we know, from previous reference already given, what kind of doctor he was, and certainly what method of treatment he used in the dressing of their wounds.

Most of the members of the Church of Jesus Christ of Latter-day Saints who emigrated to Nauvoo, were of other Sectarian faiths. In those times, it was the custom to know the Bible by heart, and often the only reading means available to many poor families was the Good Book. Such an example was the Smith family. For about the only real education which Joseph himself got, was from what he had read in the family Bible on different occasions; supplemented by only a trifle smattering of schooling, which did not amount to very much even then.

Thus, being so well versed with "the cornerstone of Christian faith," many Latter-day Saints were familiar with scriptures like:

And I, God, said unto man, Behold, I have given you every herb bearing seed, which is upon the face of all the earth; and every tree in the which shall be the fruit of a tree, yielding seed; to you it shall be for meat.

"...and thou shalt eat the herb of the field...."

So, it would only seem that the Word of Wisdom, with its strong herbal suggestion, should come natural to most of the people converted to the new faith.

But if they understood their scriptures well, then they would realize that the principles Joseph was espousing were according to the teachings of the Master Himself. Being familiar with His Words, they would understand that he often made numerous references to the herbs of the field and generously spoke about them with great frequency. And they would also know, that being a devout Jew himself, he would naturally adhere most strictly to the teachings of the Old Testament, such as those references we have examined in Genesis, for instance. His liberal use of herbs might be found sprinkled throughout his teachings and parables:

Hear ye therefore the parable of the sower.5 (A man who plants seed.)

> *And he said, So is the Kingdom of God; as if a man should cast seed into the ground; and should sleep and rise, night and day, and the seed should spring and grow up, he knoweth not how;*

> *For the earth bringeth forth fruit of herself, first the blade, then the ear, after that the full corn in the ear.*

> *But when the fruit is brought forth, immediately he putteth in the sickle, because the harvest is come.*

> *And he said, Whereunto shall I liken the kingdom of God? Or with what comparison shall we compare it?*

> *It is like a grain of mustard seed, which, when it is sown in the earth, is less than all the seeds that be in the earth; but, when it is sown, it groweth up, and becometh greater than all herbs, and shooteth out great branches; so that the fowls of the air may lodge under the shadow of it.*

> *And with many such parables spake he the word unto them....6*

It is an interesting thing to discern from the foregoing remarks of the Savior, that He considered *even* trees (the mustard tree, for example) as herbs. For, He says "when it is sown, it groweth up, and become greater than *all herbs*, and shooteth out great branches..." In the art of botanical medicine, not all herbs are considered as plants; some, in fact, come from trees, such as slippery elm, bayberry bark, etc. So, with the Savior's new interpretation upon the word "herb," it makes the explanation offered by Daniel Webster, the famous lexicographer, as given in the last chapter, much more enriched with deeper meaning. Thus, in the official use of the word "herb" in the Word of Wisdom, God is defining both plant *and tree*, as containing medicinal properties for the use and good of man.

However, the Saints in Nauvoo must have been aware that the volunteer principle upon which the Word of Wisdom was offered, coincided exactly with the Bible; and that all God was doing, was re-quoting the same thoughts of His Servant, the Apostle Paul, in different language for modern times:

Him that is weak in the faith receive ye, but not to doubtful disputations.

For one believeth that he may eat all things, another, who is weak, eateth herbs.

Let not him that eateth despise him that eateth not; and let not him which eateth not judge him that eateth; for God hath received him.[7]

This beautiful injunction, as re-phrased in modern revelation to read, "And whosoever among you are sick, and have not faith to be healed, but believe, shall be nourished with all tenderness, with herb..."[8] told the Saints how to treat one another in their respective beliefs and ideas. What Paul was saying then, was that some believed they might eat all things; but some, with not such a healthy appetite, sought to pacify their weak condition with herb dishes alone. Those who were able to eat all things, were not to look down upon those who couldn't. Or, to be more exact about the matter, the gourmet was not supposed to frown upon the one who was not, nor was the one who lacked a voracious appetite to consider the other "a pig" or "a hog." But each was to do their own separate "thing" in the best way they pleased themselves to do. And God was to be the judge of both.

For often, God would receive the one who was gluttonous, if he had lived a good, moral life upon the earth, as much as He would receive the honorable slim man, too. Here then, for the Saints was Biblical proof of what their Prophet had said. And certainly confirmed the understanding of the revelation just quoted, as detailed out in the previous chapter. For them in Nauvoo, it meant to let those who believed in herbs use them, and for those who did not believe, allow to use whatever manner of means they so desired to employ, even though it may have been contrary to Joseph Smith's own way of thinking. For, when asked upon one occasion, how he governed the people so well, Joseph replied: "I teach them correct principles and let them govern themselves." He taught the Saints to use herbal medicine:

I preached to a large congregation at the stand, on the science and practice of medicine, desiring to persuade the Saints to trust in God when sick, and not in an arm of flesh, and live by faith and not by medicine, or poison; and when they were sick, and had called for the Elders to pray for them, and they were not healed, TO USE HERBS and mild food.[8]

36

*Joseph gave a lecture on medicine. Salt vinegar and pepper given internally and plunging in the river when the tossing begins, will cure the cholera....*9

But, in no way, did he force them to use it, or compel them to. He was a Prophet, not a tyrant; a Man of God, not a dictator. His was to love and be loved; not to hate and be hated.

A Missouri minister, on visit to Nauvoo from St. Louis made the observations that he could find no trace whatsoever of any medical doctors in Nauvoo, as "the Mormon leader wouldn't allow them there." In fact, he stayed with one Mormon family just across the river, who employed the services of medical physicians contrary to the advice of their Prophet.10 Thus, we can see that not all Latter-day Saints were faithful to their Prophet's words; yet we have no evidence on record which says that God still did not love them, provided they did not apostatize completely.

The reason for which the author is detailing all of this out, in such a careful and concise manner, is that the reader may be able to realize that the aim of this booklet is objectivity. That is, to try and define things as they exactly are; but also to present a fair overview of the entire matter in discussion. For those who may be happening to read this, who are firm believers in medical science and have employed doctors over the years, the preceding material just given, states that such was not according to what Joseph Smith himself taught and believed in; yet, in no way, is it a reflection that such who believe in these things opposite the Prophet's own views, are denied the love of God because of it. They may, perhaps, be in jeopardy of disobeying a commandment, but that is not for the writer to say, one way or another. Still the fact remains, that they can and DO enjoy the love of God, though their personal opinions conflict some-what with those of Joseph Smith's. Nor does it necessarily mean that those who follow his advice on herbal medicine are especially favored of Heaven either. They only enjoy the advantage of an additional blessing by keeping the Word of Wisdom IN FULL, and nothing more besides.

Thus, we can see that God is "no respecter of persons" and will not uphold the one and deny the other. He is just as fair in His dealings with the believer in medical science as He is in the believer of herbal medicine. His Servant Joseph was this way; and certainly that fine man reflected, in a measure, by his actions the same type of a just feeling and policy which the great God above had within Himself, also.

To continue with matters in Nauvoo, though: Joseph, when sick would summon those type of men in whom he believed most sincerely:

> *Friday, December 15th, 1843. I awoke this morning in good health, but was soon suddenly seized with a great dryness of the mouth and throat and sickness of the stomach and vomited freely. My wife waited on me, assisted by my scribe and Dr. L. Richards, who administered to me herbs and—?—(smudged; unable to make out two words) milder drinks . I was never prostrated so low in so short a time before. But, by evening, was considerably revived.* [11]

Joseph Smith also instituted other means by which people could be healed and made well.

> *Early Mormon medical beliefs were strongly influenced by Dr. Samuel Thomson, not a Mormon, but a New Englander like Joseph Smith and Brigham Young and many other leaders of the Saints.*

> *Under the influence of the Thomsonians, Joseph Smith had organized a Board of Health in Nauvoo in the early 1840s.* [12]

It is needless to say, that the Board of Health which the Prophet established in the city, advocated the use of herbs and allowed for the free practice of botanical medicine, but greatly restricted others of a different profession who knew not herbs, nor the use thereof.

For those who had not faith enough in herbs, or common administrations, other measures were devised:

> *...As the congregation dispersed, I walked with the Mormon who had brought me in his canoe, to see the temple.... He showed me the great baptismal font, which is completed and stands at the centre of the unfinished temple. It rests upon the backs of twelve oxen, as large as life, and tolerably well sculptured; but for some reason, perhaps mystical, entirely destitute of feet, though possessed of legs. The layer and oxen are of wood, and painted white; but are to be hereafter gilded, or covered with plates of gold. At this place, baptisms for the dead are to be celebrated, as well as baptisms for the healing of diseases; but baptisms for the remission of sins are to be performed in the Mississippi....*[13]

He believed that the sisters should also be involved in healing the sick as much as possible. And for this reason, he gave as his opinion to the

Relief Society assembled in Nauvoo, these inspired words and kind suggestions:

> *Respecting the females laying on hands, he further remarked, there could be no devil in it if God gave His sanction by healing; that there could be no more sin in any female laying hands on the sick, than on wetting the face with water; that it was no sin for anybody to do it that has faith, or if the sick has faith, to be healed by the administration.*[14]"

The Prophet took very serious the calling of those who were to administer to the sick, and for that reason, often set many apart to that office of ministering unto the sick:

> *While living in Nauvoo, the Prophet Joseph Smith laid his hands on Ann's head and set her apart as a midwife, telling her that she would be successful in caring for the sick if she would use herbs exclusively in her work. Some years later in Utah she became known as the 'herb doctor.' She had an herb garden and prepared her own tea and medicine.*

> *When the Prophet set Ann apart as a midwife, he promised her she would not suffer at death. On July 3, 1893, she had a paralytic stroke and on the 16th of July passed peacefully away. She was 94 years of age.* [15]

> *In Nauvoo, Joseph Smith set apart three women for this calling: Vienna Jacques, Ann Carling, and Patty Sessions.*[16]

> *At Nauvoo, Ill., Dr. Calvin Crane Pendleton was set apart to care for the sick. Receiving but little income from his medical services, he earned a livelihood in his shop as a mechanic, and by his pen...*

> *Dr. Pendleton made remedies from roots and herbs that he gathered and compounded into pills.* [17]

> *My grandmother left her family, joined the Church, and walked all the way to Nauvoo. She had no place to stay and so she stayed in the Mansion with the Prophet and his family. At this time, she was only a girl of 16 or 17, I believe.*

> *The Prophet called her as 'a nurse in Israel' and set her apart for that calling. She would often accompany him on his rounds to the sick, and assist in administrations to them.*[18]

In the female meetings in Nauvoo, Illinois...midwives discussed the spiritual aspects of their work, quoting testimonies of Brigham Young and others proclaiming the blessings which had followed on the offices of mercy performed by their sisters in the calling. Since their beliefs, their customs, and the nature of their prescriptions were inextricably bound together, when they met to discuss obstetrical problems they invariably supported descriptions of unusual cases with testimonies. An extremely good example of this is Patty Sessions, one of Utah's foremost early midwives. Although she was entirely objective in her recording of medical instances and data, she was nevertheless deeply subjective as regards religion. From reading her diary one must inevitably conclude that these two attitudes were in reality inseparable. This is not the conflict of terms that it seems, if one realizes that in every venture in life these hardy pioneer women felt God's nearness and His help.

To them in Nauvoo, "God, with the all-seeing eye and the never-failing ear, was always the greatest doctor of all." When death came to a patient, it was the result of His will. Instant healing was a manifestation of His power. There was no sacrilege whatsoever in seeing a man fetch the holy oil to bless a fallen ox, or in telling that the ox, upon being blessed with the laying-on of hands, like a human being cast off his sickness through the power of God and rose to resume his burden. The Word of Wisdom, righteous living, and the use of herbs as remedies for disease and a means of sustaining health were far more important to Mormons than the "poisonous medicine" prescribed by doctors.

The great mother of Mormon midwifery, Patty Sessions, formulated these remedies for curing the sick, and used them extensively in Nauvoo:

> *Salve for old sores: Bark of indigo-weed root boiled, beeswax, mutton tallow, a very little rosin.*

> *Jaundice: Take one tablespoonful of castile soap shavings, mixed with sugar, for three mornings; then miss three until it has been taken nine mornings—a sure cure.*

> *Bowel complaint: Take one teaspoonful rhubarb, one-fourth carbonate of soda, one tablespoon brandy, one teaspoon peppermint essence, half-teacupful warm water; take tablespoonful once an hour until it operates.*

> *Vomiting: Six drops laudanum, the size of a pea of soda, two teaspoons of peppermint essence, four cups water; take a tablespoonful at a time until it stops it; if the first does, don't repeat it.*

Heart-burn: Laudanum, carbonate soda, ammonia, sweet oil, camphor. Also for milk leg inflammation or sweating.[18a]

In regards to the Nauvoo Legion, Lieutenant-General Joseph Smith allowed for only the best (as he deemed it) of skilled medicine to be used upon his military regiment. To this end then, did his personal botanic physician, Dr. Levi Richards, serve as surgeon-general to the men and treated with herbs those who were sick. [19]

In other fields of medicine, there was even a dentist in Nauvoo, who subscribed to some of the Thomsonian methods of skill and kept most of his work based on natural ingredients. He was a dentist, and this is how he advertised and worked:

> *Alexander Neibauer, the first dentist in Utah, was born near Coblentz, Prussia, January 8, 1808, son of a Hebrew physician and surgeon. Alexander was to have entered the Jewish ministry, but instead studied dentistry in the University of Berlin, beginning practice in Preston, England. While there he married Ellen Breakel, and was the first Jew to be converted to the Mormon faith; he was baptized April 9, 1838.*

> *Young Dr. Neibauer emigrated to Nauvoo, Illinois, in 1841, where he became active in the Church, and prominent in Freemasonry, while setting himself up in the practice of dentistry. He advertised as follows in the (Mormon) 'Times and Seasons,' Nauvoo, August 2, 1841: ALEXANDER NEIBAUER SURGEON DENTIST, from Berlin, in Prussia, late of Liverpool and Preston, England. 'Most respectfully announced to the ladies and gentlemen and citizens of Nauvoo as also of Hancock county general, that he has permanently established himself in the city of Nauvoo, as a dentist, where he may be consulted daily, in all branches connected with his profession. Teeth cleaned, plugged, filed, and Scurva effectually cured, children's teeth regulated, natural or artificial teeth from a single tooth to a whole set inserted on the most approved principle. Mr. N. having had an extensive practice both on the continent of Europe, as also in England, for the last 15 years he hopes to give general satisfaction to all those who will honor him with their patronage.*

> *'Mr. B. Young having known Mr. N. (in England) has*

kindly consented to offer me his house to meet those ladies and gentlemen who wish to consult me. Hours of attendance from 10 o'clock in the morning to 6 at evening.

'My own residence is opposite Mr. Tidwell, the cooper, near the water. Ladies and gentlemen attended at their own residence, if requested. Charges strictly moderate.'

He usually used a dental turnkey, an implement with a hinged claw on a gimlet-shaped handle, for extracting teeth by twisting; but he later obtained forceps. These instruments were subsequently turned over to Dr. Washington F. Anderson. Cavities in decaying teeth were cleansed with suitable picks and filled with alum and borax and then sealed over with beeswax; the only anaesthetic was laudanum. He was seldom paid in money; but accepted beet molasses, corn meal and pig-weed greens. Much of his work was donated to widows and to others who could not pay.[20]

The only exception to his practice, which did not qualify it as thoroughly Thomsonian, was in his use of laudanum, or "tincture of opium." But this he must have used sparingly, and with great caution, otherwise, the Prophet would never have allowed him to open his practice in the city, had he not attempted to subscribe to some of Joseph's beliefs along an herbal line, and thereby conduct his work the same.

Quite often in his sermons, the Mormon leader would strongly denounce the use of medical drugs. Of this historical bit, a noted writer relates the following:

In the development of both the sovereign remedy—faith healing—and the bias against 'poison pills,' the influence of Joseph Smith, founder of the Church, undoubtedly helped to shape the attitude of the society as a whole. Joseph Smith was not unlike many other religious leaders in advocating faith healing. Frequently he publicly said that he had greater confidence in its power than in any medicines or any physician who prescribed them. When addressing the Church in Nauvoo, he frankly denounced such 'poisonous medicines' as datura, henbane, calomel, and licuta stramonium...

...From Willard Richards down, the guardians of health among the Mormon people put their trust primarily in lobelia and cayenne pepper, and such herbs as goldenseal, balmony,

raspberry leaves, and sage twigs. Phineas Richards, a brother of Willard, and also a Thomsonian doctor, had a mould which turned out pills as large as horse chestnuts. These he expected people to swallow.[21]

However, some Saints who did not adhere to this philosophy of reason could get quite tacky about it, if they saw others drinking a cup of tea. To them, the Word of Wisdom was not Divine counsel to use herbs when sick, but rather a "do" and a "don't." "You do keep the Word of Wisdom, when you don't drink tea," they read it as, and maintained this line of course, no matter what may have prevailed:

Brigham may have had a latent feeling however, that diets and doctoring had a place in the Divine economy, for under the shade of the old Bowery in Salt Lake City, August 17, 1856, he had related an incident wherein Old Father Baker in Nauvoo had been called in to lay hands on a very sick sister in the Church. It was a very sickly time, and there was scarcely a person to attend upon the sick, for nearly all were afflicted. Father Baker was one of those tenacious, ignorant, self-willed, over-righteous Elders, and when he went into the house he inquired what the woman wanted. She told him that she wished him to lay hands upon her. Father Baker saw a tea-pot on the coals, and supposed that there was tea in it, and immediately turned upon his heels, saying 'God don't want me to lay hands upon those who do not keep the Word of Wisdom' and he went out. He did not know whether the pot contained catnip, penny-royal, or some other mild herb, and he did not wait for anyone to tell him. That class of people are ignorant and over-righteous, and they are not in the true line by any means.[22]

Clearly a case of where "the letter killeth, but the Spirit giveth life."[23]

Occasionally, there were some who believed that "all disease was caused by the Devil" and that "the sick ought to live by faith." For, these strange tenets of belief, they often met persecution and adversity, and sometimes even a high council trial, as the following goes to prove:

Agreeable to adjournment the High Council convened at the house of Lyman Wight on the 21st of August, 1834.

...John Corrill entered a complaint against Lyman Wight with teaching this doctrine, saying: 'All disease in this Church is of the Devil and that medicine administered to the sick

is of the Devil; for the sick ought to live by faith.' And he wished the high council to take it into consideration...

After which Lyman Wight acknowledged that he had taught this doctrine, or rather believed it to be correct.

After which, W. W. Phelps spoke and said, 'This case needs no counseling;' which was agreed to...

After which the President proceeded and gave the following decision saying: 'It is not lawful to teach the Church that all disease is of the Devil. But if there is any that has this faith let him have it to himself. And if there are any that believe that roots and herbs administered to the sick and all wholesome vegetables which God has ordained for the use of man, and if any say that such things applied to the sick in order that they may receive health, and this applied by any member of the Church, if there are any among you that teach that these things are of Satan, such teaching is not of God.

Council dismissed. Prayer by David Whitmer, President. Orson Pratt, Clerk.[24]

It is of interest to note that Lyman Wight was not reproved for believing in the doctrine, only for teaching it. The doctrine was not ruled as seditious or evil. So, it stood with a silent approval of its truthfulness—"All disease in this Church is of the Devil and that medicine administered to the sick is of the Devil..." The only emphatic injunction given against it was that such things were not lawful to teach in the Church. However, if any chose to hold to this peculiar tenet of faith, they could do so provided they kept it to themselves. The order was aimed at the individual, NOT the doctrine, as we have just seen.

Another Latter-day Saint who believed in this same thing, was Priddy Meeks. Of this doctrine, he wrote the following:

Now for those foul spirits and witches; what is the difference between them? Foul spirits are disembodied witches living in the flesh. Do they have power over human beings? They certainly do, every pain, ache, or misery we endure is attended by a spirit of affliction and that spirit is intelligence; hence, the propriety of laying on hands and rebuking it in the name of Jesus, which would be supreme foolishness if it were not intelligent...

...It is certainly fair reasoning. These kinds of spirits work mostly on the mental functions instead of the physical functions but affect the physical system unto death sometimes by tormenting the spirit of the person.[25]

The early missionaries of the Church, ever aware of the false traditions of an unbelieving generation with which they had to deal, often met Latter-day Saints who still held to the old notion and practice of medical aid, yet hoping to compromise their comfortable position with a new-found faith in God. Jared Carter was one such man, and the family whom he encountered, though members of the Church in good standing, still adhered to a belief that was not doctrinally sound, and incorrect according to Joseph Smith's teachings. Only their little boy had the common sense to see that in the one lay life, and in the other lay death. Of this circumstance, Elder Carter recorded the following:

Another manifestation of God's healing mercy took place to Brother Locke's, which was as follows—

I was there to visit them and one of their children was sick with a fever and there under the care of the doctor. This time that I was there—?—[unable to make out some words; considerably smudged]...as before that Brother Locke and his wife had joined the Church. The child was upon a bed in a room. I went to the child when alone and laid my hands upon the child and prayed that God would heal him and then I went away from there.

I, after this, went there again and found the child to appear well nigh unto death. I, on seeing that the child was worse than when I laid hands upon him and prayed for him as I thought in faith, was some considerably tried in my own mind, because the child was no better. But after hearing Sister Locke relate what took plas(c)e after I went from there, I prayed for the child as jest above-mentioned. For, she said, soon after I laid hands on the child (after I was gone) that the child got up off its own accord and came into the kitchen saying, 'Maw, Uncle Jared has cured me. Uncle Jared has made me well maw.' And she said after the child got up in this manner, she looked out and she saw that the doctor was near and had called to one of the neighbors to see one that was sick.

She, on seeing this, went down to the mill where her husband was, to see him; to have him stop the doctor from coming there; for she thought it was unnecessary that he should go there, for the child was apparently well. But her husband told her that he thought that they had better let the doctor go there, for he wanted to have the child sure to be well. The Doctor, accordingly, went there and left some medison [medicine) for the child to take. But as soon as they gave the child any more medison, the fever returned again and then the child said of his own accord after the following manner: that his Uncle Jared came there and made him well and the doctor come there and made him sick again. And the child growed (grew) worse, until I come there the second time, as above-mentioned; at which time the child, as they considered unless it was helped immediately, must soon dye (die).

But the next morning after prayer I administered the laying on of hands again. And immediately after this the child got up of his own accord and went to see his maw and said, 'Maw, Uncle Jared has made me well again.' And the child, from this time, continued well.

In this ensample, we see the impropriety of putting our trust in man; yea, the impropriety of disobeying the command of God as unto the church; wherein, he has required of this church, that they would not employ physitions [physicians) of the world....[26]

A very clear piece of evidence to show "the impropriety of putting our trust in man; yea, the impropriety of disobeying the command of God as unto the church...." And the requirement set down by God Himself that "this church...WOULD NOT employ physitions [physicians] of the world...."

Those who are raised with the belief to trust in medical doctors, should realize what the Prophet Joseph Smith said about such traditions, in the light of modern revelation upon those matters:

I say to all those who are disposed to set up stakes for the Almighty, You will come short of the glory of God.

To become a joint heir of the heirship of the Son, ONE MUST PUT AWAY ALL HIS FALSE TRADITIONS.[27]

And, it can be safely assumed that whatever traditions we cling to, which may conflict with the Gospel of Jesus Christ, then those traditions must be wrong. For, it is man's puny thinking against the judgment and wisdom of God, and who can dare gainsay the difference between them as to which one is better? Error must always bow out when truth steps in, or else progression—both mortal and immortal, halts.

Inasmuch, as the Saviour made reference to herbs often in His Sermons, and the Prophet Joseph Smith sought to emulate the Master's life in every respect, even to the inclusion of herbal medicine in his way of living, then it would be a good thing to remember this, in closing:

For thrones, dominions, kingdoms, powers,
And glory great and bliss are ours
If we, throughout eternity,
Obey His words, ' COME, FOLLOW ME!' [28]

IN SUMMARY

1. The noblest message which can be given to mankind by Jesus Christ, is the simple phrase: "COME, FOLLOW ME!"

2. Jesus often made many references to herbs in His Sermons and Parables.

3. The Apostle Paul had a modified version of the Word of Wisdom for his time.

4. Joseph Smith emphatically preached herbal medicine to the congregations assembled often in Nauvoo, to hear their great leader speak.

5. A Gentile visitor discovered the absence of medical doctors in Nauvoo.

6. When Joseph Smith was sick he allowed only herbal physicians to attend him.

7. An Herbal Board of Health was established in Nauvoo, under the direction of the Prophet.

8. The Gentile visitor discovered that they performed baptisms for diseases in the font of the Nauvoo Temple.

9. Joseph Smith said that women could lay hands on the sick and heal them, too.

10. Joseph Smith believed that nursing and tending the sick was important enough to make it a religious calling in the duty of faith, and promptly ordained and set apart all those whom he called to this great service to the Saints at large.

11. The Nauvoo Legion was attended by an herbalist in times of sickness.

12. Nauvoo had its own Jewish dentist who practiced along some of the lines of herbal faith.

13. Joseph Smith strongly denounced drugs in their rudest form.

14. To believe that "all disease" is "caused by the Devil and that "all medicine administered to the sick is of the Devil" is not a sufficient complaint enough to call wrong or false; but strong enough to prohibit from making it a church doctrine in public.

15. Priddy Meeks, a reliable Latter-day Saint practitioner, sincerely believed that evil spirits were the cause of "every pain, ache, or misery we endure.

16. False tradition is hard to do away with, in any form.

17. God has commanded the Church not to employ physicians of the world, according to the sober statement of Elder Jared Carter.

18. Joseph Smith said that we must put away our false traditions, or we cannot inherit the Celestial Kingdom as a God or Goddess.

19. If we are to have eternal glory, we must obey His words,

"COME, FOLLOW ME!"

CHAPTER FIVE

LOBELIA—THE CORNERSTONE OF HERBAL FAITH

(A Description and Short History of the Most Popular Herb in Mormon Medicine)

Joseph Smith had this to say about the plant now in discussion:

Dec. 26th, 1842. Visited Sister Morey in custody of Lee (?) and prescribed for her afflictions; spoke very highly of Lobelia. Good in its place. Was one of the works of God. But like the power of God or any good, it became an evil when improperly used. Had learned the use and value by his own experience.... [1]

When the Prophet had suggested the use of this herb, he was recommending one of the finest plants known to man. To acquaint the reader with "the most powerful relaxant known among herbs" but one which leaves "no harmful effects,"[2] the following short description is furnished for the reader's information:

LOBELIA

(Plant and Seed)

Botanical Name: Lobelia inflata. Coninon Names: Blader podded lobelia, wild tobacco, emetic herb, emetic weed, lobelia herb, puke weed, asthma weed, gag root, eye-bright, vomit wort. Medicinal properties: Emetic, expectorant, diuretic, nervice, diaphoretic, antispasmodic.

... Lobelia acts differently upon different people, but it will not hurt anyone. It makes the pulse fuller and softer in cases of inflammation and fever. Lobelia reduces palpitation of the heart. It is fine in the treatment of all fevers and in pneumonia, meningitis, pleurisy, hepatitis, peritonitis, phrenitis, hephritis, and perositis. Lobelia alone cannot cure, but it is very beneficial

49

if given in connection with other measures, as an enema of catnip infusion morning and evening. The enema should be given even if the patient is delirious. It will relieve the brain. Pleurisy root is a specific remedy for pleurisy, but it is excellent if combined with lobelia for its relaxing properties. The use of lobelia in fevers is beyond any other remedy. It is excellent for very nervous patients. Poultices of hot fomentation of lobelia are good in external inflammations such as rheumatism, etc. It is excellent to add lobelia to poultices for abscesses, boils and carbuncles. Use one-third lobelia to two-third slippery elm bark or the same proportion to any other herb you are using.

While lobelia is an excellent emetic, it is a strange fact that given in small doses for irritable stomach, it will stop spasmodic vomiting. In cases of asthma, give a lobelia pack, followed the next morning by an emetic. The pack will loosen the waste material, and it will be cast out with the emetic. In bad cases, where the liver is affected and the skin yellow, combine equal parts of pleurisy root, catnip and bitter root. Steep a teaspoonful in a cup of boiling water. Give two tablespoons every two hours, hot. For hyrophobia, steep a tablespoonful of lobelia in a pint of boiling water, drinking as much as possible to induce vomiting. This will clean the stomach out; then give a high enema. This treatment should be given immediately after the person is attacked. Lobelia is excellent for whooping cough.... There is nothing that will as quickly clear the air passage of the lungs as lobelia. A tincture made as follows will stop difficult breathing and clear the air passages of the lungs, if taken a tablespoonful at a time:

Lobelia herb	2 ounces
Crushed lobelia seed	2 ounces
Apple vinegar	1 pint

Soak for two weeks in a well-stoppered bottle, shaking every day. Strain and it is ready to use. This is also good to use as an external application, rubbing between the shoulders and chest in asthma. Lobelia poultice is excellent for sprain, felons, bruises, ringworm, erysipelas, stings of insects, and poison ivy.

An associate of the Prophet Joseph Smith's, relates a healing incident involving the use of this wonderful herb with a patient of his in Nauvoo, and describes some of the virtues of this plant in general:

*Sister Daniel Tyler, while living in Nauvoo, got desper-
ately poisoned by rubbing red precipitated mercury on her skin
for the itch, not knowing the danger. She put it on quite plentiful.
He came for me about midnight. I just gave her a few courses of
Thomsonian medicine, and it was not long before she was well.*

*We need to know but little about the patient, only to
know that they are sick; and but very little difference what the
complaint will be, thorough courses of regular Thomsonian
medicine will seldom if ever disappoint you in performing a
cure. It will remove obstructions wherever found in the whole
system and restore a healthy action wherever needed. It does
act like intelligence, always in harmony with the living intention of the system which is always to remove obstructions from
the system of whatever name or nature it may be.*

*I sometimes look upon lobelia as being supernatural
although I have been using it for forty-six years. I do not know
the extent of its power and virtues in restoring the sick and at
the same time perfectly harmless. It is undoubtedly the best and
purest relaxum in the compass of medicine. That is the reason it
is so good in childbed cases; it puts the system exactly in the
situation the laws of nature would have it be to perform that
object. Those in the habit of using it in such cases look forward
in pleasing anticipation of having a good time, without fore-
boding of trouble so common to women. Oh glorious medicine!*[4]

Priddy Meeks testifies concerning lobelia in this fashion:

*...a sure, quicker, and more powerful anti-poison (I
think), is not known, and probably never will be.*

*As an instance, I attended a case of hydrophobia. A boy
ten or twelve years of age, Philetus Davis, by name, having been
bitten by a rabid dog, lobelia was administered. He recovered
perfect health, and says he has never had a tremor of the
complaint. He now lives in Toquerville, and has a large family.*[5]

Another instance of its unique properties may be seen in this
recorded manifestation:

*Brother Nobel's wife, within about one month of her
expected sickness, had the dropsy so bad he thought she could
not live until that month was out, so that she could be doctored
without injury to her offspring. The doctors in the valley had a*

consultation over her case, and President Young with them; they could devise no means to save the woman without destroying the infant and she could not live but a few days without help; but they would not make a move until they sent for me. When I came they told me they could not see how the woman could be saved without destroying the child. I told them there would be no difficulty in bringing about that object. They wanted to know if I thought that I could take the water out of that woman and save both alive. I said, 'Yes, I certainly can, and lobelia is the thing that will do it.' I just gave her Thomsonian courses of medicine and soon had the water all out, and in due time she had a fine boy to the joy of all who were watching to see what the result would be.[6]

To most herbalists of the Mormon faith, in practice then, this plant was "the cornerstone of their faith." One of the most active of botanic physicians, Priddy Meeks, looked upon it this way:

I don't know what encomiums I could place on lobelia to be competent with its virtues, the extent of its therapeutic action on the human system. I think there are but few if any who understand. I have been in the habitual use of it now for forty-seven years and I don't profess to know all about its operations on the system yet, neither do I ever expect to until I understand the physiology of the human system more than I do and the laws of which it is governed, for lobelia will act on the system in complete conformity with the laws of health; and when that law is obstructed and fails to fulfill the operations that nature intended it to fulfill while healthy, it will remove those obstructions wherever located, for lobelia will permeate the whole system until it finds where the obstruction is seated and there it will spend its influence and powers by relaxing the parts obstructed.

There should always accompany the lobelia with cayenne pepper which is the purest and best stimulant that is known in the compass of medicine. It will increase the very life and vitality of the system and give the blood a greater velocity and power. Now the system being so relaxed with lobelia and the blood being so stimulated with such power it will act on the whole system like an increased flow of water turned into a muddy spring of water; it will soon run clear and although lobelia is set at naught and persecuted the way it is, it is for the same reason that the Latter-day Saints are persecuted; IT IS

ORDAINED BY GOD TO BE USED IN WISDOM. *The world will not persecute them that are like them, but hold them the same as their own.*7

It was with great frequency that the Latter-day Saints used and employed lobelia; for it was "the cornerstone" of Thomsonian medicine and the chief herb around which all others revolved. Men such as Dr. Frederick G. Williams, Dr. Willard Richards, Dr. Levi Richards, Dr. Calvin Pendleton, Priddy Meeks, Patty Sessions, and other skilled botanic physicians, did not hesitate to recommend this important herb, nor stress its vital significance in the practice of their art. We suppose countless volumes could be written of the times it was used, and hundreds of pages consumed in recording all of the marvelous experience connected with this Divine creation. But one should suffice for now:

> *Another incident I will relate while I was cutting up the lap of a large oak tree, together with a man named Jackson, as it was our day to work tithing. We were strangers to each other. It was hot weather and very sickly. Some would take the fever and die before the news would get circulated. Early in the day he suddenly took a very high fever; it was a very serious case and he was very much alarmed about it. I told him that there was a little weed growing around I thought might do him good. He eagerly wished for it. It was lobelia of the first year's growth. Some not much larger than a dollar and lay flat on the ground. I got some of it and told him to eat it, just like a cow would eat grass and he did so, and in a few minutes it vomited him power-fully and broke the fever and he finished his day's work. I mention this to show you what virtue there is in lobelia.*8

Sometimes there was even an added bonus to the virtues of this herb; like a Heavenly visitation, for instance:

> *In this connection I will relate another visionary inci-dent while living at Parowan. Simeon Houd got badly poisoned with strychnine, so that he had to have his thumb amputated, but that did not seem to stop the poison from ascending up his arm and going down into his vitals which would prove fatal. He sent for me and said to me: 'Brother Meeks, if you cannot save me I am gone; for if the poison gets into my vitals it will kill me; it is now to my shoulder.' Never knowing lobelia to fail in a case of poison, neither indeed in any other case, in full assurance of faith, I went to work and gave him several thorough courses of Thomsonian medicine, and in three or four days he was so much*

better that we all believed that nothing more was needed as the poison was checked; he felt about well. I thought the job was completed and I went home.

The second night after I went home, a strange young woman dressed in white appeared to me and said, 'I am sent from the other world to tell you that if you do not double your diligence on Brother Houd he will die, for Satan is trying to kill him.' I said, 'Did you say that you came from the other world?' 'Yes,' she replied. 'Do you know anything of Calivin (sic) Smith, who was President at Parowan and has been dead about a year?' 'Yes, I came from where he is.' I said, 'How is he getting along?' She said, 'First rate; but he is mighty busy.' 'What is your name?" said I. She said, 'Sally Ann.' But the other part of her name I either forgot or did not understand; I could not repeat it in the morning. She said she had two cousins here and wanted to visit with them while she was here. I asked her their names. She said, Julia Thompson and Sarah Smith, both daughters of Horace Smith Fish, who lived in Parowan.

I said to her, 'You must not be out of my presence while you are here; (that order was given to me by inspiration), but I will tell you how we can do. I will go with you and then you will be with me all the time.' It was known to me instinctively that I was responsible for her while she stayed here. So we both went to where each woman lived but did not get an interview with either of them, but the cause I did not know. There was something dark about, and I went back to my house. She said, 'Now come with me; I want to show you a pretty building.' We entered the beautifullest building that I ever saw. It was spotless white inside. It needed no candle to give light. It was unfurnished, no furniture or anything else in it. She said nothing about who would enjoy the building. She showed me several rooms or departments all exceedingly beautiful. Now said she, 'I am ready to go,' and I said, 'Go.' And soon as daylight I went to Brother Houd. I doctored him about as much as I had done, taking the same course I had done before and he was soon well and lived about twenty-five years afterwards.

So when I told Sisters Thompson and Smith, what she told me about being cousins they said, 'We know who it was.' It was Sally Ann Chamberlain who died fourteen years ago at their home not far from Nauvoo. I mentioned the interview we tried to have with them. They both said they were troubled that night and could not sleep and thought that there was someone there who wished to see them and got up and lit a candle and searched the house, and went out of doors and looked around but could see no person. Now from this woman I learned two important facts. One is when a messenger is sent to anyone they are responsible for them as long as they are with them. The other was that the principles I aim to doctor on are correct. If it had not been so, she would have to change my course instead of telling me to double my diligence. 9

Some even enjoyed certain visions in the night, portraying this herb as the standard for all that was good:

Mrs. Ferris closes by quoting Sister Sessions, who related a dream in which she witnessed a remarkable fight between the Lord and the Devil—the Devil almost won the fight— the moral or conclusion of which was 'THE LORD ADVISED HER TO USE LOBELIA in curing disease, as that would drive the Devil away.' 10

However, at times there could be dissensions in the ranks, and what would be considered one man's medicine, was thought by another to be his poison:

Austin N. Ward was a guest of Mr. Hinckly at the Social Hall, where at least sixty-five women were present. Dr. High spoke attributing disease to the violation of physical laws. Dr. Speight dissented in many particulars, believing that sickness was often sent by Divine providence. Sister Newman also opposed some of Dr. High's theories and was sure God sent many afflictions. Sister Lippincott recommended catnip tea; but Sister Gibbs is alleged to have declared catnip tea was good for nothing; said enough lobelia would drive all the devils out. Mr. Ward, obviously relishing the experience, says Mrs. Gibbs in a frenzy, spoke in tongues, and afterward fell asleep. Sister Sanders expressed her firm belief that all diseases could be cured by faith and the laying on of hands; and Sister Petit told of a dream in which the Devil fought God. —Ward's narrative is so similar to Mrs. Ferris' narrative one wonders which is hearsay and if either is history![11]

However, the scope of this disagreement is fully realized, when one considers the tremendous explosion which erupted between two herbal doctors of divergent views. One believed in using lobelia as an emetic, and would swear by it to his dying breath; this was Dr. Meeks. The other man was somewhat inclined toward surgical practices found in the medical profession of those times; this was Dr. Pendleton; and the issue resolved itself this way:

> *My wife, Mary, gave birth to a daughter about 10 PM (Sunday). The infant was rather small, but well, weighed 6 1/2 pounds. Everything did not work right with my wife. The nurse gave her an emetic [lobelia] which threw her into spasms. These spells lasted about 36 hours, having one every hour. She was insensible all the time. They put hot rocks on her to steam her and burnt her feet and legs so bad that quite large pieces came out. The whole ball of one of her big toes came off from the burn. Dr. Meeks was called in; afterwards Dr. Pendleton. They did not agree in their methods of treatment. Pendleton finally had her bled in the ankle to bring the blood from her head. Meeks got mad at this and left. He was quite stubborn about the case. Brother (Arrzasa) Lyman (an Apostle) called the case up in Council and reprimanded Meeks for his course. Lyman spoke about it in public meeting.*

> *So the doctor was criticized by the priesthood because he did not believe bleeding at the ankle to draw blood from the head would aid a woman recovering from childbirth.* [12]

In commenting upon the above-related circumstance, the author will only say this: Whoever administered the lobelia to that poor suffering woman, should have remembered Joseph Smith's injunction about its use —— "[lobelia] good in its place...but like the power of God or any good, it became an evil when improperly used." Too much of anything no matter how good it may be, can be harmful and sometimes, lethal also. As for the high council trial of Brother Meeks, it seems that a man's stubborn attitude was labored beyond just a mere shrug, and that some parties involved felt to make a case of the issue.

Another severe account on record, in which lobelia was employed, and with which happy results were met, is the following:

> *Barnabee Carter got struck with a piece of cast metal drum in a machine that was going a furious speed. It burst all to pieces, one piece went through the weather-boards of a house that stood some distance off. One piece or two struck Carter on the breast and side and knocked him down with a dangerous wound. Being unconscious, he was carried home. There was a*

great excitement, very warm water, and a great crowd. There was no gash cut, but a terrible bruise and it was turning blue. I told them I wanted them to leave and give me a chance and I would promise them there should not be left a blue spot of bruised blood under the skin in a short time. In this case I gave lobelia as well as cayenne pepper to relax the system so that the bruised blood would assimilate with the warm uninjured blood and become equalized through the whole system. I don't know that I gave lobelia enough to puke him or not. If I did it was so much better. [13]

It should here be noted that, perhaps, one cause of the difference which existed between two of Utah's most prominent doctors—the lobelia specialist, Priddy Meeks, and the herbal practitioner, Calvin Pendleton—may have been jealousy. You see, both men lived in the vicinity of Parowan, Utah. Pendleton lived right in the townsite itself, and Meeks lived a ways out. Maybe the vying for potential customers on both parties was one reason for this jealousy between them. Anyhow, they did not get along very well together.

To conclude this chapter, we offer the humble statement of Priddy Meeks himself in relation to lobelia—the "herb of herbs:"

I do not think the medicine is yet found and probably never will be that will act in accordance with the laws of life and the intention of nature like lobelia. No difference what the matter is or where the obstructions are, lobelia will find it and remove the obstructions and create a healthy action. On, wonderful medicine that will act, so much like intelligence; but cayenne pepper and sweating ought always to accompany a course of medicine; and also an injection (enema). [14]

IN SUMMARY

1. Joseph Smith advocated the use of lobelia.

2. Lobelia is good for many things. It is an excellent remedy for someone who has been bitten by a rabid animal. It settles the stomach in small doses, and relieves it up in larger doses. It is an excellent bowel mover, when accompanied with cayenne pepper.

3. It is the best antidote against internal poisoning known to man.

4. It Is a wonderful aid in pregnancy, when administered WITH SKILL.

5. According to one of the greatest users of it in Mormondom, Priddy Meeks: "IT IS ORDAINED BY GOD TO BE USED IN WISDOM."

6. A Divine Being appeared to Priddy Meeks and urged him to DOUBLE his efforts in the use of lobelia upon a sick and dying man.

7. Patty Sessions, a faithful Latter-day Saint was ADVISED BY GOD TO USE LOBELIA IN ALL OF HER PRACTICES.

8. Even herbal doctors do not agree on some things together.

9. The wonderful virtues of lobelia cannot be extolled enough.

CHAPTER SIX

THE WAYS OF HEAVEN—REVELATION AND HERBS

(Faith-Promoting Incidents of Inspiration in Mormon Medicine)

Because most of the early Latter-day Saints came from an early American or English background, it would only stand to reason that most had been subjected to one form of Sectarianism or another; and some, perhaps, to quite an extent. Be they Baptist, Methodist, or Church of England, it would be logical to assume that a lot of them were acquainted with their Bible quite well. If we stop for a moment and analyze the actions of young Joseph Smith, we will realize that he turned immediately to the Bible after hearing a sermon preached by a Sectarian minister in his parents' church, which he happened to attend one Sunday. And, of course, that scripture in James led him to the great religious experience which he had later on in the Sacred Grove, some distance from his home. Thus, we can see from this little incident how extensively the Bible was relied upon and used by people then.

It seems that as a general rule, more of early America in those primitive times, were intimately acquainted with what the "Good Book" said, than are people today in this country. People had more of a religious attitude toward things then, and a reverence and respect borne of Bible indoctrination, than what presently prevails among our citizenry.

Being so closely connected with the Bible, in almost every aspect of their lives, these early converts to the new faith of Mormonism would, of necessity, know how God felt toward doctors, from what they read, or did not read. A learned commentator on the Bible put it this way:

> In the Old Testament, there is little place for the physician, if indeed, he existed at all, because God alone was regarded as the healer. He was the source of life and health, sending disease and disaster to Mankind as punishment for sin; and healing it only if the sufferers were worthy of cure. 'If thou wilt

diligently hearken unto the voice of the Lord thy God, and wilt give ear to His commandments, and keep all His statutes, I will put none of these diseases upon thee which I have brought upon the Egyptians; for I am the Lord that healeth thee.' (Exodus 15:26)

Any human knowledge of healing was regarded with disfavor, lest it should attract from a power which ought to belong to God alone. Few remedies are mentioned in the Old Testament, and in every case the treatment is recommended by a 'Man of God.' Naaman, the leper, is told by Elisah (2 Kings 5:10) to wash himself seven times in the River Jordan; King Hezekiah, 'sick unto death' from a boil (the exact diagnosis is obscure) is bidden by Isaiah to apply a lump of figs (2 Kings 20:7); while Elijah restored to life the son of the widow of Zarepath, apparently performing artificial respiration (I Kings 17:17-18).

If physicians did exist among the Jews when the Old Testament was written, there is surprisingly little reference to them in the sacred writing. The oft-quoted eulogy, commencing, 'Honor a physician with the honor due to him for the uses which ye may have of him; for the Lord hath created him,' is from a book, which, strangely enough, was not included in the Canon, The Wisdom of Jesus, the son of Sirach or Ecclesiasticus.[1] It is a noble testimonial to the medical profession, although the last verse, 'He that sinneth before His Maker, let him fall into the hand of the physician'—is capable of more than one interpretation. [2]

Thus it would only be proper to admit that most Biblically-minded Latter-day Saints would not employ the use of doctors but rather rely upon faith and inspiration to do the healing work for them. A fine example of this may be found in Mother Smith's own family. Her oldest brother, Jason Mack, was an inspired man of God, before the introduction of the Restored Gospel, and enjoyed such benefits and blessings as them who believe, receive. He was a standard for good wherever he went, proclaiming the gospel as he understood it from the Bible, and healing the sick by the laying on of hands, as well as the ministration of mild herbs and such unto them. In all of this, he moved as he was conducted to do so by the Spirit of the Lord, and did it all in the name of Jesus and good faith, without any priesthood means whatsoever. This is not to imply, however, that priesthood is not necessary; for surely, he must have been limited in the amount of good which he could have done otherwise, had he had the

Melchizedek Priesthood with which to operate by. Nevertheless, such as what he did enjoy was the means of great comfort and much security to those unto whom he ministered. An account of this goes as follows:

> *Jason...became what was then called a Seeker, and believing that by prayer and faith the gifts of the gospel, which were enjoyed by the ancient disciples of Christ, might be attained, he labored almost incessantly to convert others to the same faith. He was also of the opinion that God would, at some subsequent period, manifest his power as he had anciently done—in signs and wonders...*

> *...'according to my early adopted principles of the power of faith, the Lord has, in His exceeding kindness, bestowed upon me the gift of healing by the prayer of faith, and the use of such simple means as seem congenial to the human system; but my chief reliance is upon Him who organized us at the first, and can restore at pleasure that which is disorganized.*

> *'The first of my peculiar success in this way was twelve years since, and from nearly that date I have had little rest. In addition to the incessant calls which I, in a very short time had, there was the most overwhelming torrent of opposition poured down upon me that I ever witnessed. But it pleased God to take the weak to confound the wisdom of the wise. I have in the last twelve years seen the greatest manifestations of the power of God in healing the sick, that, with all my sanguinity, I ever had declared with sober face, time and again, that disease had obtained such an ascendency that death could be resisted no longer, that the victim must wither beneath His potent arm; I have seen the almost lifeless clay slowly but surely resuscitated, and revived, till the pallid monster fled so far that the patient was left in the full bloom of vigorous health. But it is God that hath done it, and to Him let all the praise be given.*

> *'I am not compelled to close this epistle, for I must start immediately on a journey of more than one hundred miles, to attend a heavy case of sickness; so God be with you all. Farewell*

> *'Jason Mack'*[3]

Now, in the book of Isaiah, we read the following familiar piece of scripture:

> *For my thoughts are not your thoughts, neither are your*

ways my ways, saith the Lord.

For as the heavens are higher than the earth, so are my ways higher than your ways, and my thoughts than your thoughts.

Now, one of the peculiar tenets to Mormon belief, is that every man might enjoy for himself, distinct revelation from on High. No other religion in the world makes such a bold and definite claim of the matter as we do. And, because of this unique privilege enjoyed by every worthy Latter-day Saint man, woman, or child, they ought to be able to receive for themselves the correct manner of things they need, in which to go.

Such, then, is what the Lord has promised His Children that if they would become His People, then He would lead them in the paths of righteousness forever!

The early period of the Church was fraught with much hardship and social ills. People were often left in dire predicaments and desperate situations, from which the only recourse seemed to be: turn to God and trust in Him, with all 'heart, might, mind and strength.' And when they did so, they found Him to be there when they needed Him and required His Services. And found Him to be the same loving God which He has always been; and discovered for themselves, this testimony: that indeed, His ways are better than man's ways.

Willard Gilbert Smith was the son of Warren and Amanda Barnes Smith. He was born May 9, 1827, in Amherst, Lorain County, Ohio, and was the eldest child in a family of eight. Willard's parents joined the Church of Jesus Christ of Latter-day Saints early in 1831, just one year after the Church was organized...

On the morning of October 30th, they arrived at a little place called Haun's Mill, a small settlement on Shoal Creek, composed of Latter-day Saints...

...'Myself and two brothers were with father when, without warning a large body of mounted men, blackened and painted like Indians, rode up yelling and commenced shooting at the crowd.

'The men at the shop called for quarters; to this the mob paid no attention. The men then called for the women and children to run for their lives.

'We were surrounded on three sides by the mob; the old mill and mill pond were on the other. The men ran for the shop, taking the little boys with them. My two little brothers ran in with father. I followed but when I started to enter the shop my arms flew up and braced themselves against each side of the door, preventing my entrance...I ran around the corner of the shop and crawled into a pile of lumber, hiding as best as I could...

'As soon as I was sure they had gone, I started for the shop...I said, 'Alma is alive but they have killed father and Sardis'.... Mother leveled the straw, laid some clothes over it and on this...we placed Alma, and cut his pants off. We could then see the extent of his injury. The entire ball and socket joint of the left hip was entirely shot away, leaving the bones three or four inches apart. It was a sickening sight, one I shall never forget. Mother was full of divine, trusting faith, a most marvellous, wonderful woman.... Mother said, 'All right, let's pray to the Lord and ask Him (what to do).' So we all gathered around him on his bed of straw and mother prayed, dedicating him to the Lord, asking God to spare his life if He could make him strong and well but to take him to Himself if this were impossible.... In her terrible excitement and sorrow, her only help seemed her Heavenly Father. So she prayed for guidance, pleading for help in this dire extremity. By inspiration her prayers were answered and she knew what to do. She placed little Alma in a comfortable position on his stomach, telling him, 'The Lord has made it known to me that He will make you well, but you must lie on your stomach for a few weeks.'

'Mother was inspired to take the white ashes from the campfire, place them in water to make a weak lye, with which she washed the wound; all the crushed bone, mangled flesh and blood were thus washed away, leaving the wound clean and almost white like chicken breast. Then she was prompted how to make a poultice for the wound. Mother asked me if I knew where I could get some Slippery Elm tree roots. I said I knew where there was such a tree. She gave me a lighted torch of shag bark hickory with which to find my way.

...I took the torch and ax and soon got the roots from which mother made a poultice, with which she filled the wound. As soon as the poultice turned dark it was removed and the wound washed and re-filled. 5

63

From this beautiful story we learn that the Lord was able to inspire this woman with the right kind of method for treating her son, and able to show this to her through the fine medium of revelation.

Such Divine wisdom and inspiration even attended the Prophet Joseph Smith at times when he was sick. For, we find in one recorded instance, that his attendant felt impressed to do nothing but give him enemas during the entire course of his fever:

> *The Prophet at this time sick with the fever, chose me as his constant nurse and companion, and I will here say, as a valuable hint to the wise, that the sanitary treatment of copiously flushing the colon with water, much upon the present 'Hall System,'*[6] *was about his only remedy.*[7]

And a missionary in the Church from Nauvoo, while in the field earnestly performing his assigned labors, found himself in such a literal "scratch" of things, that it required Divine guidance again, to remedy his excruciating suffering:

> *...'I caught the itch, which nearly cost me my life. An Elder that traveled with me on one occasion, advised me to get some mercury, dissolve in water and wash wherever I was broken out with this rash, which I did, in a cold room; which caused it to strike inwardly.*

> *'I was very sick the day I done this. I had to travel about 16 or 17 miles and hold three meetings. I got through, but oh my, it was a hard day's work.*

> *'The Spirit of the Lord suggested to me to get some burdock roots and make some tea and drink it freely, which I did, and it killed the effects of the mercury, and I recovered.'*[8]

And during the hard days experienced at Winter Quarters, the suffering Mormon pioneers found they had very little to subsist upon. "They had not food enough to satisfy the cravings of the sick, nor clothing fit to wear. For months thereafter there were periods when all the flour they used was of the coarsest, the wheat being ground in coffee and hand mills, which only cut the grain; others used a pestle; the finer meal was used for bread, the coarser made into hominy. Boiled wheat was now the chief diet for sick and well. For ten days they subsisted on parched corn." As the scanty food supply was getting dangerously low, some felt inspired to mix "their remnant of grain with the pounded bark of the slippery elm which they stripped from the trees along their route."9 Thus, was an otherwise unpalatable meal, made somewhat nourishing and healthy by the addition of this fine herb.

In the trying times of tested faith, when "the famine had waxed sore" in the Valley, and the plague of the crickets came, many families were without meal, or flour, or any kind of grain with which to make bread. It was here that the Lord provided for them to eat the "bitter herb of the field" for survival.

Beef, milk, peg-weeds, segoes, and thistles formed our diet. I was the herd boy, and while out watching the stock, I used to eat thistle stalks until my stomach would be as full as a cow's.

Even when there were no herbs around to subsist upon, or mingle with other scraps of food, or to remedy a physical complaint, revelation afforded other means, such as prayer, by which a man could be benefited:

I often suffered with acute, cutting pain in my stomach, which at times would cause the sweat to start from every pore. This, with constant piles and tendency to dyspepsia, made me very unfit for such arduous labors. The duties alone of caring for the teams and other camp duties looked great indeed to me, and coming from one of the best tables in Nauvoo, with my delicate appetite—now how was I to live!

After being a few days in camp, some commenced to complain of hardship and poor fare, but President Young roared upon them like a lion, and told them, and all who could not then commence to live upon 'boiled beans and corn,' trust in God, and be grateful for what they did get, should start back at once, for the camp of the Saints would be a poor place for them. This came to me as the word of the Lord, but what was I to do?

For a long time I had been unable to eat cornbread or beans, as they gave me those unbearable stomach pains, how could I then go, for the most we had now for food was corn and beans. I felt it was a subject of life or death to me, and I asked myself what show there would be for me in turning back with my three wives; and whether it were not better to die, trusting in the Lord and being faithful than to feel that I could not conform to the necessities of the journey and go forward.

This was on Sunday, and in the evening, we talked the

matter over. I told my wives I was there to trust in the Lord, and if He was not with us He certainly was not behind us, and I should not go back. I was willing to eat such food as we had and be grateful for. And if the Lord did not take care of us now; the sooner we were all dead, the better, for we would not be able to care for ourselves or protect our lives upon this journey.

...And here I will say that before breaking camp at Sugar Creek, the beans and corn, formerly uneatable by me, I could eat with relish, and from that time the old effect did not return to me on the journey. I had told the Lord what His servant had said, that by His help I would fulfill every requirement, and if it was His will that I should live to be His servant, He must cause my food to assimilate to the condition of my stomach, which I know He did. [11]

Now to many of us in modern times, such simple remedies of herbs and plants might seem all a bunch of bunk. What God would consider a plant of great virtue, man may think of as a weed, and trample it beneath his feet. A noted herbalist, who had a genuine appreciation for the finer things of life, had this to say about the blossomed creations in Mother Nature:

When I study the herbs, flowers, roots, barks, and the leaves of the trees, and see the wonderful medical properties they contain, the marvelous benefits that are derived from their use, I feel that the word 'wonderful' is inadequate to express the real truth. The phrase, 'the mighty miracle working power of God' is none too strong. If you had seen the things that have actually been done by the use of these herbs in connection with hygenic measures, you would not think for one moment that these statements are overdrawn. As I go out into the woods and see the lofty trees, I feel like taking off my hat in reverence to God for the wonderful medical properties in these various trees for the healing of man as well as for their use for building houses in which to live, furnishing fuel with which to cook our food, and heat to keep us warm. [12]

And so it was, that God in His great, infinite wisdom sought to raise the lowly, despised thistle into a category of respectability, by revealing its "manifest destiny" to the mind of one Latter-day Saint, through revelation:

June 3, 1864. Received a beautiful letter from my father.

After describing the suffering he had endured lately from an attack of liver complaint, he says, 'On Saturday last I went to the South Mountain to seek the face of my Physician and to pour out my complaint into His ear where none but He could hear. I asked Him to relieve me of my distress or voice of my mouth and by His Holy Spirit enlightened me to know that He had stored up virtue in the noxious thistle, exactly suited to my disease, and as it was before me I gathered it, brought it home, stewed it up in water, ate it and found relief. Blessed be the name of Him who lives from age to age without change.' [13]

Often the men of herbal medicine were inspired by revelation, too:

He and I were digging potatoes one evening and it was not time to quit work yet, an impulse struck me to look toward Cedar City; we could see the road five or six miles distance, and and when I looked I saw the dust rising in the road. The impulse struck me again with force as much as to say, 'There is someone from Cedar City wanting you to go there to doctor someone, and now cover up your potatoes with vines to keep the frost off.' 'Come Dick,' I said, 'let us cover up our potatoes.'

We had just finished and met the messenger at the field gate some two or three hundred yards from the house, saying, there was a woman at Cedar City that would die before morning without assistance, so I went. The woman had a rising in her breast which was expected to break inside any minute which would prove fatal; but by making an incision with a lancet two inches deep it reached the corruption and she was instantly relieved, and was soon well.

My course in general has been AN INSPIRED COURSE *all through my life.*

Priddy Meeks, the botanic physician of Southern Utah, often received unusual, though true, doctrine with regards to his practice, by that penetrating influence which leaves no doubt:

May the 19th, 1882. This morning a few thoughts forcibly suggested themselves to me before I got out of bed. Old people that have passed the turn of life should not eat much cold victuals nor take heavy draughts of anything that is cold because they are deficient in the warmth of the system and what little warmth there is in the system has to be assimilated into the cold that is in the system to bring the temperature of the whole system into an equilibrium; this instead of increasing the heat (which is one great object in eating), it decreases it. Heat is life or the residence of it and the more warmth until it comes to the maximum of health the more life is enjoyed and (vice-versa). The more cold the more death, till warmth is overpowered and the life goes out with the warmth.

All men and women are subject to this law because they all pass through the turn of life, similar (no difference) and that consists in passing down the stream of life to mingle with their native element and that turn of life consists in the drying up of the nervous system. The calves of the legs become flabby and loose like a cow's bag half milked and every muscle, leader and tendon in the whole system becomes weakened and relaxed. It certainly is supreme reasoning that the very life of man can be cultivated and improved and lengthened out on the same principles as other things and I believe that the improvement would be just as great in man as on Irish potato or the lower order of animals. Isaiah says in the last chapter, but one: That the days of man shall be as the days of a tree. And it is reasonable to suppose that his physical power will develop and increase according to his longevity.

All this will be brought about upon common sense principles, and when we learn common sense principles in taking care of ourselves and practice it and take common sense remedies and eat common sense food, eating nothing that will militate against our health, wear nothing that will militate against our present or future comfort, take no medicines that will poison the system and adhere to the Word of Wisdom that says, all wholesome herbs are ordained of God for the constitution and nature and use of man and then practice it, then will the human family begin to lengthen out their days, longer and longer as they practice those principles till the days of man will be as the days of a tree; not suffering the ravages of sickness and misery that now afflict the present generation in consequence of their not observing the laws of health and longevity and keeping the commandments of God.

Then will the powers of the priesthood become more of a supreme fact in the eyes of the nations of the earth in controlling foul spirits and the spirits of disobedience. Although the devil *will be close on our heels as long as he can muster his forces to come up against the Saints of the Most High God. But there must be an opposition in all things and let us prepare ourselves for it by dealing justly, and loving mercy and walking humbly before our God.*[14]

Before we close this chapter, it will be necessary to look at another phase of herbal medicine in Mormonism. And this has to do with the use of olive oil within the Church of Jesus Christ of Latter-day Saints. The lexicographer, Mr. Webster, considered the olive tree a thing "of antiquity." When one searches the oldest Book known to man, he readily comes to find out just how true this is.

The reason we have to classify olive oil with herbal medicine, is because it figured in with certain other herbs in times past:

Among all the ancient Eastern nations, olive oil was one of the most precious of products. It was used lavishly by the Egyptians for their hair and the skin, as well as in all sorts of ceremonies.

To the Israelites in the Desert, the anticipation of the 'corn and wine and oil' of Canaan was always present, and throughout their history there are abundant evidences of how they prized it.

The prescription for the 'holy anointing oil' given in Exodus, xxx, 23, is very remarkable. It was to be compounded of the following ingredients:

Flowing myrrh	*500 shekels*
Sweet cinnamon	*250 "*
Sweet calamus	*250 "*
Cassia (or costus)	*500 "*
Olive oil	*One hin*

A hin was a measure equivalent to about 5 1/2 of our quarts. The shekel was nearly 15 lbs., and some of the Rabbis insist that the 'shekel of the sanctuary' was twice the weight of the ordinary shekel .[15]

As can be clearly seen, the other above ingredients are all herbs, which were to be mixed together with pure olive oil and made into "a confection after the art of the apothecary."[16]

In modern times the "symbol of peace" has had its oil used for purposes besides cooking. In the field of general medicine, the use of olive oil has been strongly recommended by some prominent medical men in such diverse ways as "an enema consisting of four ounces of olive-oil" given for obstinate constipation.[17] And this, too, advised by a man who was a member of the American Medical Association, the Chicago Medical Society, and Superintendent of the North Yakima (Washington) General Hospital. [18]

And a nationally-recognized dietician of the 1920s, Dr. Frank McCoy, found olive oil indispensable in the eradication of gall stones from the system:

> *The first method of treatment to be used for any disorder of the liver or gall-bladder is the olive oil and fruit juice regime. Just before retiring, the patient usually takes 4 ozs. of olive oil, together with 4 ozs. of lemon, orange, or grapefruit juice. The oil and fruit juice are beaten up well together into as much of an emulsion as possible, and the mixture, if taken just before retiring, is less liable to cause nausea while the patient is asleep. This may be taken on one night only, or on several nights in succession, and should be followed by a fast with grapefruit juice, lemon juice, or orange juice. This fast should be continued as long as necessary, and the olive oil treatment may be taken as many times as seems advisable to accomplish a thorough cleansing of the gall-bladder and liver...*

> *Case 45. Man, 40 years of age. Had suffered from several attacks of gall-stone colic, and had been advised to undergo an operation, but would not consent, because in several cases with which he was familiar where operations had been performed, the patients had only received temporary relief, and after-wards had a more aggravated form of the trouble than before.*

> *I was called in on the case while he was having a most severe attack of gall-stone colic, and it was several hours before the cramps could be relieved. At first he was so nauseated that everything taken into his stomach would be immediately vomited, and the olive oil regime could not be administered until after the acute attack had subsided. However, through the use of small amounts of lemon juice, together with hot applications*

*over the gall-bladder and hot enemas, the trouble was suffi-
ciently relieved during the first day to enable him, after 24 hours
of this treatment, to retain 4 ozs. of olive oil and 4 ozs. of lemon
juice. After taking these, he was able to sleep for 12 hours, being
utterly exhausted from the acute attack.*

*As soon as he awakened he was given an enema of 2
quarts of hot water. This brought away about 200 small gall-
stones with quantities of bile and mucus. The olive oil treatment
was administered each night for three more days, the patient
using a lemon juice fast during the rest of the time, that is, taking
the juice of half a lemon in a glass of water every half-hour of the
day. The fast was not continued long, as the patient wanted to
get back to his office for some important business, so he was put
upon a careful diet, and the olive oil and grapefruit juice taken
every third out with the enemas until they were all gradually
eliminated, and at the end of 30 days there was no further sign
of anything except bile being brought away.*

*This cure was effected over four years ago, and the
patient has remained in perfect health ever since, with not the
slightest return of any symptom of gall-stones. He has also
remained well in every way, without any of the headaches which
he experienced for so many years, and which were no doubt
caused by a chronic state of biliousness.*[19]

These uses of olive oil were not just confined to the Gentile popu-
lace alone. In fact, at one time in Mormonism, it used to be quite the thing
to take consecrated olive oil internally, as part of the general good medicine suggested by God. Saints thought no more of consuming it internally
as they did of drinking herbal teas, and felt that it was as proper and right
in its place to take as botanic medicine was. One recorded instance of this,
where the person felt to relieve himself of doctors and trust in God, is:

*About the first of the year, 1852, Thomas was taken
suddenly ill with bilious fever and brought home for treatment.
The father very much against the wish of Thomas, sent for a
doctor, who attended him for five or six weeks without any sign
of improvement; in fact, he continued to grow worse. The father
became greatly alarmed and discouraged, lest he also should
die.*

*Finally, Thomas determined to have his own way in the
matter of remedies, and the next time the doctor called he told*

him he had decided to take no more of his medicine, and to dispense with his services. He asked his father to throw away all of the doctor's medicine that he had, and to get him a bottle of olive oil, and he would take that and trust in the Lord for the result.

He took about half of the bottle of oil, which caused nausea, and he really felt for awhile as if he was dying, but after vomiting very freely, and thus relieving his system of a good deal of the poison which had accumulated therein, he felt better and from that time improved.[20]

Another case on record, wherein olive oil was connected with a marvelous spiritual manifestation, is this:

My mind reverts back a few years when I had a little sick girl on Thanksgiving, who was not expected to live. She was fighting for breath, and to live seemed impossible. Yet from the very beginning she had faith that she would live, and what made her so firm about it was that she, in the dreariness of those long nights of affliction, had a vision. A personage appeared to her, clothed in white, standing as it seemed in the air; and he brought to her bedside such peace and joy as none can describe or express. This made her say within herself, 'I know I am going to get well.'

This little girl was what you would call an invalid for two years, notwithstanding she was prayed for constantly by relatives and friends, and she saw the good of prayer. Many times was she relieved of pain instantly by her own prayers and also by the prayers of the Elders of the Church. One day she said: 'Ma, how I wish I could go to the temple! I know I should get well.' And she prayed earnestly that she might go.

One day a sister by the name of Hjorth, who now lives in Fairview, heard of it and sent word that she was going to the temple and would be glad to take the child with her without expense—for us just to prepare her clothes and send her to her. In a few hours she was off, for it so happened that her clothes were in readiness. She was gone ten days and our family fasted and prayed for her the day we thought she would be in the temple, and the little boys expected to see their sister healed instantly.

But God saw fit for us to wait yet a little longer. She came home rejoicing and telling how she cried when she was blessed, though she couldn't tell why she was crying. She said, 'Ma, there was the sweetest feeling there! How earnestly they prayed, and they promised me I should get well. If I could always feel like I did there, I would not care if I had only a crust to eat.'

This was in the Manti Temple. When she came home she brought a large bottle of oil with her and worried much for fear it would not last till she got well, for she thought she couldn't get any as good as that. But she got well in six weeks, had some of the oil left, and is now strong and healthy. She has worked and has earned her mother a new dress for this Thanksgiving, which caused her to shed tears of joy, and to feel to thank God for the blessings He bestowed upon her child.[21]

In closing, it would be good to keep in mind that revelation is the object which fills the gap of human ignorance, and supplies man the knowledge he needs at that time. And also to remember, the words of a well-known Mormon hymn:

GOD MOVES IN A MYSTERIOUS WAY

God moves in a mysterious way,
His wonders to perform;
He plants His footsteps in the sea,
And rides upon the storm.
Deep in unfathomable mines
Of never failing skill,
He treasures up His bright designs,
And works His sov'reign will.
His purposes will ripen fast,
Unfolding every hour;
The bud may have a bitter taste,
But sweet will be the flower.
Blind unbelief is sure to err,
And scan His work in vain;
GOD IS HIS OWN INTERPRETER
AND HE WILL MAKE IT PLAIN. [22]

IN SUMMARY

1. The Bible has little use for physicians, and any healing done therein, is automatically attributed to God.

2. In ancient times, Men of God often advised the proper medicinal remedy to employ in cases of sickness or illness.

3. Jason Mack, an uncle to the Prophet Joseph Smith, enjoyed inspiration while healing people.

4. God's ways are higher than man's ways.

5. A woman with a mortally-wounded child, was inspired by the Holy Ghost, the proper manner in which to treat him, and the right herbs to use also.

6. Joseph Smith believed in flushing the colon with water when sick (or taking an enema, to be more practical about the subject).

7. A missionary received revelation from God to use a certain herb with which to relieve himself of a terrible itching sensation.

8. When hungry the pioneers often would be inclined to eat of the herbs of the field, when food was scarce and in short supply.

9. Faith and prayer relieved a stomach condition.

10. The wonderful medical properties in trees and plants are indescribable.

11. Something so common and despised as the lowly thistle, even has virtue in it!

12. Revelation can bring some good, sound principles on general health to a person, if they are desirous of learning more in that direction.

13. In ancient times, olive oil was used in conjunction with other herbs.

14. The healing properties of consecrated oil, when taken internally, are not to be underestimated.

CHAPTER SEVEN

THE MORMON LEADER WHO VACILLATED

(Brigham Young and the Doctors)

The position of Brigham Young in regards to medical doctors is a rather difficult one to state. On the one hand, he followed closely behind the martyred Seer and Revelator in the same footsteps which Joseph had walked. On the other hand, he seems to have been inclined away from herbs somewhat, toward a more practical acceptance of medical science at the close of his life. For quite a while he seemed to maintain Joseph's ethics and beliefs in relation to the medical profession at large. As early as 1846, we find him issuing the following statement to the Mormon Battalion:

> Camp of Israel, Omaha Nation
> Cutler's Park
> August 19th, 1846

> *To Captain Jefferson Hunt and the Captains, Officers, and Soldiers of the Mormon Battalion.*

> *We have the opportunity of sending to Fort Leaven-worth this morning by Dr. Reed a package of twenty-five letters, which we improve, with this word of counsel to you all:* IF YOU ARE SICK, LIVE BY FAITH, AND LET SURGEON'S MEDICINE ALONE. IF YOU WANT TO LIVE, USING ONLY SUCH HERBS *and mild food as are at your disposal. If you give heed to this counsel, you will prosper; but if not, we cannot be responsible for the consequences. A hint to the wise is sufficient.*

> *In behalf of the Council,*
> *Brigham Young, President.[1]*

Willard Richards, Clerk.

It would seem from this that President Young was as strongly influenced against these things as what his predecessor had been. Hence, the imparting of this advice to the men. However, they were under a different type of command—a Federal one, officered by unprincipled men of the United States Government, who insisted—nay, demanded, absolute loyalty under any circumstances. And with their caravan was a wicked Missouri doctor, who hated the Mormons with a passion. His name was Sanderson, and "he threatened to cut the throat of any man who would administer any medicine without his orders."[2]

Now, Brigham Young had counselled privately with Col. James Allen (the recruiting officer of the Battalion) in matters of the utmost concern governing the volunteers from the Mormon encampments. Among other things which he discussed with Col. Allen was the necessity of having a good botanic physician along to treat the people of their faith, with the things they believed in.[3] Hence, we find a Mormon herbalist, one Dr. McIntyre, accompanying the men along on their journey.

This is officially set down in a direct order issued by the army colonel while at Fort Leavenworth:

HEADQUARTERS, MORMON BATTALION,
COUNCIL BLUFFS,
July 16, 1846.

(ORDER No. 3)

William L. McIntyre, of the Mormon people, is hereby appointed assistant surgeon to the Mormon Battalion of volunteers of the United States, and under my command. He will be obeyed and respected accordingly, and will be entitled to the pay and emoluments as an assistant surgeon in the United States Army.

J. ALLEN, Lt. Col. U.S.A.,
Commanding.[4]

Despite this legal confirmation, we find the following problem developing after the unfortunate demise of such a good man:

Dr. McIntyre, a good botanic physician, had been appointed assistant surgeon by Colonel Allen on the day of our enlistment; yet under pain of this threat he must not administer one herb to his afflicted friends and brethren unless ordered so to do by the mineral quack who was his superior in office.[5]

Such resentment was there expressed toward the unjust treatment they received under this medical doctor's hand, a parody was composed by Levi W. Hancock, entitled "The Desert Route," which set down in two verses their precise feelings upon the subject of men and medicine:

> *A Doctor which the Government*
> *Has furnished, proves a punishment!*
> *At his rude call of 'Jim Along Joe,'*
> *The sick and halt, to him must go.*
> *Both night and morn, this call is heard;*
> *Our indignation then is a stirr'd,*
> *And we sincerely WISH IN HELL,*
> *His arsenic and calomel!*[6]

It is an amazing fact to consider that some eight years later, the smoldering anger these men felt toward Dr. Sanderson, became alive and was renewed at a gathering of the Battalion in Salt Lake City, February, 1855. Perhaps no more resentment has ever been kindled in the hearts of the Mormon people toward medical doctors, as it was toward this old mobocrat. The toasts which were offered in behalf of this man's unworthy name, went as follows:

> *Captain Brown: 'Here's to all oppressors of the Mormon Battalion; may they wither as the leek, and be carried by the Devil, and become servants to the Battalion and their children to the latest generation.*
>
> *Here's hoping old Dr. Sanderson's profession in the future state may be giving calomel to our enemies in hell. Amen!* —*T. S. Williams*[7]

Brigham Young's attitude remained quite definite for a number of years in relation to the medical profession, in general. We find that shortly after the Saints had become established within the Valley,

> *A doctor from Illinois wrote to Brigham Young to volunteer to bring a large group of neighbors to Utah as converts to Mormonism. Brigham told him that if he wanted to earn his bread like an honorable man he would be welcome, but that there was VERY LITTLE NEED FOR DOCTORS IN UTAH.*[8]

President Joseph Young, Brigham's elder brother, speaking in the Tabernacle, January 3, 1858, re-echoed the same strong sentiments which his brother felt about medical men, only in a modified sense, though:

> Paul says, 'The law of life in Christ Jesus has made me free from the law of sin and death.' Life and liberty are connected together. I sometimes visit the sick. Says I, 'What is the matter with you?'

> 'O, I am sick.' 'What is the cause?' 'I do not know.' 'Are your stomach and bowels regular?' 'No.' 'Have you taken any medicine or used any measures to remove this disease?' 'No I thought I would send for the Elders for I do not believe in the doctors; I would rather call upon the Lord.'

> Let us look at this thing. There is a class of people here that do not believe in sustaining professional doctors. I am one of them. There is a certain class of people, again, in this community, when they are sick, the very first motion they make is to call upon a doctor as quick as possible. Which of these two classes are right? Neither of them. I will not say that I would not send for a doctor in some instances, for example, to perform some difficult surgical operation, if I knew he was a good surgeon; then there are instances of sickness in which I would not send for a doctor, because I understand the nature of the disease and know how to treat it, as well and better, perhaps, than any doctor, and, aided by the blessing of the Lord, I can check it, and that is my duty. But, if I have the Spirit of God dwelling in me, my tabernacle is not very apt to be diseased.

> 'But,' says one, 'I am diseased all the time.' You may have brought your disease into the world with you, or from the country from which you have immigrated, and coming into a healthy climate, as this is, you feel the disease moving about in your system and it sometimes appears in a form which you call the erysipelas.[9]

About this same time, we find the first indications of the great Mormon leader's vacillation from one extreme to another. In the brief statement provided below, we find that while he is not challenging medical science, he certainly is not advocating herbalism, either. Rather, he is insistent upon maintaining a happy medium between them both. Looking at it from a practical standpoint, he observed:

If we are sick and ask the Lord to heal us, and to do all for us that is necessary to be done, according to my understanding of the Gospel and salvation, I might as well ask the Lord to cause my wheat and corn to grow without my plowing the ground and casting in the seed. IT APPEARS CONSISTENT TO ME TO APPLY EVERY REMEDY THAT COMES WITHIN THE RANGE OF MY KNOWLEDGE, and to ask My Father in Heaven, in the name of Jesus Christ, to sanctify that application to the healing of my body.... It is my duty to do, when I have it in my power. Many people are unwilling to do one thing for themselves in case of sickness, but ask God to do it all.

Now this pronouncement of his is certainly worthy of a little consideration as we examine the prevalence of herbal medicine in Mormon history. Brigham Young was a practical sort of a man; and while not entirely relying on the "arm of flesh," yet he was for combining all of the science and skill known to man, and applying it for the good use and benefit of the Saints in general. Thus, he may have encouraged home manufacturing on the one hand, and yet on the other, he and his associates founded and established Zion's Cooperation Mercantile Institution (or better known today as just Z.C.M.I.), which was a Mormon-sponsored department store, carrying Gentile goods from the East. Another good example was the coming of the railroad to Utah. He viewed it in two lights: one, as a good thing for the Saints, because it would make the transportation of granite blocks from the stone quarry in the mountains, to the Temple much easier. Two, it was a bad thing, in the sense of the riff-raff it would bring in with it; i.e., Gentiles from all parts of the country. Yet, from the practical standpoint he allowed it, because it would be a means of conveying God's Work that much faster to the people (speed up the building of the Temple for vicarious work to be done therein).

Here then, we have the beginnings of a situation developing in Mormonism that was to continue for some years until the death of this man; and that is, his fluctuation from the one to the other. Because in 1875, just two years before his demise, we find him again reasserting his old Nauvoo-Winter Quarters-early Valley beliefs, in this manner:

It is God's mind and will that they (every father and mother) should know just what to do for them (their children) when they are sick. Instead of calling for a doctor you should administer to them by the laying on of hands and anointing with oil, and give them mild food and HERBS and medicine that you understand.[11]

Where then was the "supposed" Mind and Will of God in the matter? Here then was a Prophet speaking, or God's Own Mouthpiece declaring the Will of Heaven to the people, or, at least that's what it was intended to be anyway.

This critique is not prepared from the viewpoint to castigate the Mormon leader for his vacillation; but rather to offer a logical explanation for his seemingly inconsistent views at the time offered on the subject in discussion.

Brigham Young is not an easy man to figure out. For example: In Nauvoo he was the sole means of saving Orson Pratt from committing suicide by jumping in the river. Orson had been somewhat despondent over the affairs of his unruly wife and his unhappy relationship with the Prophet Smith, from false accusations tendered against the man by Mrs. Pratt. As a result, he had brought these charges against the Prophet, and refused to be reconciled in the matter, even when clearly shown that his wife had told a bare-faced lie; and that the real culprit was John C. Bennett. Orson would not forgive the Prophet, and so he was cut off the Church.[12] These sad affairs and other brooding thoughts led him to take a fateful walk down to the river one day; and it was only Brigham who intervened and was the means of saving his fellow apostle from a very foolish act.

And yet, we find later on in the Utah period, Brigham severely chastising Orson Pratt on several different occasions. One was in the book Orson published entitled, "The Works of Orson Pratt," which was a series of pamphlets composed by him over an extended period of time. A certain tract in particular was called "The Great First Cause," in which this apostle espoused the belief that all self-moving particles of the universe were individual entities of intelligence, governed by their own free system of movement. This Brigham could not go along with, as the theory did not jive with his own reckonings on the matter. Thus, we find upon one occasion some rather nasty remarks made by him in rebuttal to this notion:

Sunday meeting at Beaver, Utah. President Young spoke. He spoke his feelings in great plainness concerning O. Pratt and his publications. He said Orson Pratt would go to Hell... 'He would sell this people for gold. What would I give for such an Apostle; not much and yet we hold him in fellowship in the Church.'[14]

This is not meant to serve as a discussion of other items, nor to wander away from the general theme of the subject at large; but merely to introduce a circumstance of interest, to show how contradictory Brigham Young could be in his feelings and views at certain times. Hence, in the early part of his ecclesiastical career we find him quite adamant in his feelings against medical doctors. However, toward the close of his long reign of leadership, we find that he has become more and more inclined toward the practice of general medicine in Utah, and less influenced by the botanic arts so long in existence then.

An observation has been made that:

in the first ten years of Utah settlement it is probable that most of the medical treatment was of an herb nature, with a few patent drugs that might be brought in by those who went east on a mission or to bring in a company of pioneers. 15

It was during this period and even on into the 60s, that President Young felt the necessity of employing only botanic physicians and midwives who would minister nothing but herbs. In fact, so strong did he feel about it, that he maintained the precedent which Joseph had set in Nauvoo by calling certain women to these vital positions, ordaining them, and setting them apart for that purpose.

Eliza R. Snow came to Richmond to find two women to be sent to Salt Lake to study midwifery. I, Sarah Jane Lewis and Mrs. Sarah Durney were chosen. When I found I was to go, I said plenty of mean things about the ones who thought I could go. I was leaving nine children, the youngest 18 months old. I thought there were plenty others who could go easier and do better work than I. My sister Julia, wife of Henry Grow lived in Salt Lake City, so I decided to go with her and have a heart to heart talk with President Young and tell him how impossible it would be for me to leave my family. President Young listened to me very patiently and then said, 'Sister Lewis I will give you my blessing—you will stay here the allotted time, study—your children will be well and happy during your absence. You shall be blessed in your work. When you have a difficult case, call on me, I promise to be with you, and above all, have faith.'

On returning home I had the best of luck. I always lived in settlements where there were no doctors until Doctor Adamson came to Richmond in 1893. I not only attended women but doctored men and children and was never sorry for the knowledge I attained. I always thought of myself as a missionary.

It appears that the young woman (Sarah Jane Lewis) had an undying faith and confidence in the blessing of Brigham Young. From the practice of obstetrics she branched into other phases of the roll of 'country doctor.' The large portion of the rest of her active life she spent caring for the sick. She was always subject to call, day or night. Most of her work she did as a matter of free service. Occasionally a patient was able to pay and when she could, Sarah Jane's 'going price' was three dollars for a delivery. Never did she receive more than five dollars. In the summertime she would gather tansy, horehound, peppermint, rhubarb-root, and sage, dry and powder them, and place them in her small black satchel along with calomel, assafetida, camphor, etc. [16]

And another small reference to a different mid-wife he called later on:

Sara LaDuc Pope had a natural aptitude for nursing and although she had never received special training, Brigham Young recognized her ability along this line and set her apart as a midwife and nurse.[17]

Though few are aware of it, there was at one time in Utah an herbal council of botanic physicians, apparently a carry-over of the same type of thing Joseph Smith established in Nauvoo in the early 1840s. This group was named the Council of Health, and as their parent Council of Health in Nauvoo had been, was founded and based by Thomsonian doctors upon Thomsonian principles of herbal medicine. Priddy Meeks was the one responsible for organizing it, and writes of its birth in the following manner:

The second winter we were in the valley, Apostle Willard Richards wintered in a wagon by a foot stove alone. I frequently visited him for a social chat which was very interesting to me. I learned many interesting truths from him.

Doctor William A. Morse was a faithful laborer among the sick with me, and a very good man. He and Brother Phineas Richards (another man) and myself were engaged among the sick. We had but little time for ourselves, viewing the situation of so much sickness. I proposed to my two partners in medicine,

Brothers Morse and Richards, for us to form some kind of an association for giving information to the mass of the people in regard to doctoring themselves in sickness so as to help themselves and lighten our burdens.

So we three went into the wagon to Apostle Richards and made known our wishes on the subject and he approved of it very readily and we formed a society. And Apostle Richards named it the Society of Health. We had a good deal of chat on the subject pro and con and the spirit of union was in our midst and we had a precious time of it. So much so that the Spirit impelled Brother Richards to prophesy that those principles that we were about to publish to the world would never die out or cease until it had revolutionized the earth. That declaration was an impetus to me that is in my breast today. They saw fit to appoint me President of the Institution. We conducted everything by majority.

They chose Doctor Morse and myself to scour the canyons every Wednesday in search of roots and herbs to present to the Council on the next day, Thursday, which was our meeting day for inspection and investigation of what we would bring in. It was a speedy way to become acquainted with the flora of the country and the virtues and properties of each plant for which Dr. Morse was the most famous. The masses of people then began to profit by it because of the knowledge they had gained to know what to do, as the prejudice of some people always goes in advance of every good work. It was so in this case.

A certain woman made light of the meeting to another woman. So the second woman would not go to the meeting because the first woman spoke lightly of it. One of her children took sick and died. After that she thought she would go to the Council of Health and see and hear for herself, and while there the case of her child was so plainly illustrated and how to cure such cases she remembered it and sometime after that she had another child taken with the same complaint the first child died with, and she cured it by following the directions she heard in the Council of Health. Now it was remarkable that no two canyons afforded the same kind of plants altogether for we found something new in each canyon.

The institution was so beneficial and so successful that the public began to be universally interested in it. Old Dr. Cannon, a poison Doctor, and poisoned against the Mormons too, could get but little to do among the sick; said if we would give them all the surgery to do he would quit doctoring, and so we did and he joined the Council of Health and proved a great benefit to us, being a man of much experience and intelligence. I learned considerable by helping him to dissect the dead. And after I moved to Parowan in 1851, President Young visited Parowan. I asked him, 'Has the Council of Health died a natural death or what has become of it?' He said: 'It will never die, as long as you are living.' I believe he had knowledge that I was born for that. [18]

The *Journal History of the Church* makes mention of this council twice within a short period of time:

February 21, 1849: 'Willard Richards had a medical conference in his wagon in the afternoon; similar meetings had been held during the past three or four weeks.'

A month later the same exhaustive history source, maintained by the Church Historian, Willard Richards himself, quoted the "History of Brigham Young" as follows:

President Willard Richards informed me by letter that the Council of Health had selected me and President Heber C. Kimball members thereof, and Presidents ex-officio; and also stated that Dr. William A. Morse was delegated to confer with us on the expediency of...visiting the large island in the Great Salt Lake...for the purpose of...securing for medical purposes, such saline plants and roots as were much needed.

Dr. William A. Morse announced in the first number of the Deseret News (founded June 15, 1850), by the Church; Willard Richards, (editor) that the meetings of the Council of Health were being held every two weeks at the house of Dr. W. Richards:

...Though we may fail to convince some of the superiority of the botanic practice, we feel confident that our exertions, under this head, will shake the faith of many in the propriety of swallowing, as they have long done with implicit confidence, the most deleterious drugs.... We intend to lay before the Council from time to time, such medicinal plants as shall come to our

knowledge, for their approval or refusal, as we shall find in this vicinity; believing in the goodness of the Creator that He has placed in most lands medicinal plants for the cure of all diseases incident to that climate, and especially so in relation to that in which we live.

According to the *Deseret News* of September 4, 1852, the Council of Health was held in the Tabernacle on August 31, 1852, addressed by Prof. Albert Carrington. He spoke on the relations between husband and wife, in the interests of a healthier posterity. There are other references to the Council, one in much detail being given by Mrs. B. G. Ferris in "The Mormons at Home," p. 199. While Mrs. Ferris was obviously quite as interested in discrediting the Mormons as in displaying her own superiority, her report, stripped of its sarcasm, may be of interest:

I attended a meeting of the Council of Health yesterday. This is a sort of female society something like our Dorcas Societies, whose members have meetings to talk over their occasional aches and pains, and the mode of cure. There are a few who call themselves physicians, and they are privileged to a seat in this important assemblage. The meeting was in one of the Ward school houses. There were from forty to fifty present, old and young. The meeting was called to order by Dr. Richards, hoary headed, whose looks were sufficiently sanctified to remind you of some of our good deacons at home. A Dr. Sprague, then rose and made a few commonplace remarks about health. As soon as Dr. Sprague sat down, Sister Newman said that Mormon women ought not to be subject to pain, but that disease and death must be banished from among them. She was succeeded by Sister Susanna Lippincott. She advocated pouring down lobelia until the devils were driven out of the body. Sister Gibbs got up, fully possessed, to overflowing, with the notion of healing, even to the mending of broken limbs, by faith and the laying on of hands. By some unlucky mishap, her arm had been dislocated, and she roundly asserted that it had been instantaneously put into its place by this divine process. [19]

During the territorial days of Deseret,[20] when the only tolerance Brigham had for the medical profession was in good botanic physicians, these men practiced widely throughout the valleys. The majority of their methods used seemed to be within the bounds of Divine Wisdom and good, common sense. However, a few of their techniques could be considered a little strange, and sometimes bordering on the ludicrous. One such down-right funny practice was employed by Dr. Morse, a mentor of the

Council of Health and a competent herbalist in other ways, but questionable in this instance:

> Wm. R. Palmer relates the following incident, told to him by David Bulloch as a personal experience. Mr. Bulloch, then a young man residing with his parents in Cedar City, had been desperately ill for a week with abdominal cramps and a severe pain in the right side—doubtless appendicitis.
>
> Home remedies had failed to give relief and the anxious parents sent post haste for Dr. Morse.... Galloping the twenty miles on relay mounts, Dr. Morse arrived in the nick of time—dispersing a flock of chickens as he dashed into the Bulloch doorway.
>
> 'Dave,' said the doctor, gravely, after a thorough examination, 'if it's inflammation of the bowels, I think I can cure you; but if it's mortification, all the doctors in Hades can't save you!' Ordering a live chicken caught, the resourceful doctor split it wide open and pressed the bloody bird, still squirming and squawking against the patient's bare abdomen. This was continued, with relays of chickens, as fast as they cooled, all through the night. The pain subsided by morning, and in a few days, young David was going about his work, completely healed. 'Thank the Lord it was only inflammation and not mortification,' observed David, through the memory of years; 'But I was a bloody mess, and the bed and the room looked like a slaughter house after a busy day!'[21]

But the Council of Health seemed to continue in pretty good health otherwise, save for an occasional member "chickening out" as has just been related. The *Millennial Star* of September, 1852, published the following article:

> Arrival of Mails from the Great Salt Lake valley. We have received Deseret News to the 26th of June, letters, etc., from the Salt Lake Valley.
>
> The Council of Health assembles frequently. Members continually increasing. The Deseret News remarks: 'An increased desire for the promotion of health is manifest, particularly among the ladies of the Council; and propositions are now up for improving the fashions in dress, which will tend not only to health, but happiness, comfort, ease, beauty, and every-

thing that is delightful in female economy, and gentility... Great exertions are made by the sisters to prepare themselves to nurse. Each good man will lend his influence and aid to accomplish this object, regardless alike of personal aggrandizement, and pockets full of gold.

The members of the Council, together with many of the citizens, left Salt Lake City on the 16th of June, and held a picnic on the top of Ensign Hill, where they were addressed by Patriarch John Young and James W. Cummings.

The Council of Health was established to devise ways and means to prevent disease, etc., and for preparing and administering of herbs and mild foods to the sick, according to the holy commandments of God.

Sometime in the late Winter and early Spring of 1856, the President of the Council of Health, Willard Richards[22] took very sick with the dropsy[23] and was confined to his house. During this period of time, his young stripling son, Heber John waited patiently upon his father. With his slight frame, dark eyes, and somewhat detached manner, yet with his probing, insistent mind, the tall lad had proved to Willard a constant reminder of his deceased wife Jeanetta. The youngster would often ask his beloved father, "Pa, may I bring your slippers? Will it ease your pain if I rub your hand and arm?" Dr. Richards had always had poor circulation throughout his entire life, and suffered terribly during the cold spell on the plains while at Winter Quarters. As his remaining weeks ticked slowly away, the boy was constantly by the ailing man's side, ministering unto him whatever comforts he could. Frequently he would light the apostle's pipe at the hearth and take it to him.[24] Finally, however, the end came, and Brigham Young's Second Counselor, breathed his last and passed away in peace. Naturally, he had a botanic physician by his side, when he went. This was his own brother, Dr. Levi Richards.[25]

It was whispered in some circles that the Council of Health would end, now that its President had succumbed. But following the death of Dr. Richards, this article appeared in the Deseret News:

...by desire of the late Prs. Willard Richards, and urged thereto by repeated solicitations from many of the sisters, it is my intention on or about the 1st of May (1855) to open classes for instruction on the principles of midwifery and the management of women and children. The course of study will comprise two distinct series of lectures, one designed especially for the benefit

of the matrons practicing midwifery. The other, of more general application addressed to 'Mothers in Israel' concerning the management of women during pregnancy, lying in and nursing; and also the treatment of infants and young children...the entire series to consist of sixth lectures...examinations will take place at stated period during the course on midwifery, and at the close certificates of proficiency will be granted accordingly. The introductory lectures will be delivered free at the meeting of the Universal Scientific Institution in the Council House, on Saturday evening, April 21, 1855, on which occasion the times and places of delivering the subsequent lectures will be announced.

William France, Surgeon. [26]

Toward the close of the year 1869, we find the great Mormon leader, Brigham Young still unchanged in his views toward medical doctors, when he sternly admonished the Saints in the Tabernacle, on November 14th:

Learn to take proper care of your children... If any of them are sick, the cry now, instead of 'Go and fetch the Elders to lay hands on my child,' is, 'Run for a doctor...you should go to work to study and see what you can do for the recovery of your children. If a child is taken sick with fever, give it something to stay that fever or relieve the stomach and bowels, so that mortification may not set in. Treat the child with prudence and care, with faith and patience, and be careful in not overcharging it with medicine. If you take too much medicine into the system, it is worse than too much food... It is the privilege of a mother to have faith and to administer to her child; this she can do herself.[27]

It was only in the beginning of the 1870s that Brigham Young's inclination toward doctors and the medical profession became intensified, terminating in acute. Though he delivered several good strong sermons reminiscent of earlier days, yet his leaning back the other way toward that which he had once abhorred was quite definitely evident. In tracing this through, we must keep in mind some of the scientific developments in those times, which pushed Gentile medicine significantly ahead toward twentieth-century enlightenment. A few of these notable discoveries were:

In 1837, James Y. Simpson introduced chloroform; Joseph Lister taught antiseptic bandaging.

In 1847, the American Medical Association was organized, and for the first time a national movement to improve the quality of medicine was initiated. Also, to effectively replace the Thomsonian System of Cure which was highly popular and very extensive in America then.

In 1849, Addison described pernicious anemia and suprarenal disease, a syndrome thereafter known as Addison's Disease.

In 1850, Daniel Drake published his first book on the diseases of the Mississippi Valley.

The year 1851 saw Helmholtz invent the ophthalmoscope.

The Crimean War of 1853-56 led Florence Nightingale into the founding of modern nursing.

In 1855, Claude Bernard discovered the vasoconstrictor and vasodilator nerves.

The period of 1846 through 1860 saw ether anesthesia come into general use.

In 1861, Pasteur discovered anaerobic bacteria, an event which led to the introduction of antiseptic surgery by Lister in 1867. The use of antiseptic surgery permitted operations never dreamed possible before.

The year 1876 saw the founding of John Hopkins University, in which was America's first graduate school.

In 1880, Pasteur isolated streptococcus and staphylococcus. The same year the American Surgical Association was founded.

In 1882, Koch discovered tubercle bacillus, followed by discovery of cholera bacillus in 1884.

In 1886, Fits described the pathology of appendicitis.

Finally, in 1893 Roentgen discovered the X-ray. By the

time Utah became a state in 1896, medicine was well on its way toward its present greatness.[28]

By the time the 1870s had rolled around, there had been enough important advances in medical science to warrant Brigham's attention and notice. He viewed these, possibly, as he viewed the railroad, and felt that by their inclusion into Mormon society, the people of God would stand to benefit all the more. Hence, we find him in 1872 calling his nephew, Seymour B. Young (son of his brother, Joseph W. Young, who was opposed to medical practitioners) to be a doctor and sent him off to New York City to the College of Physicians and Surgeons, now a part of Columbia University.[29] In 1873, Brigham called the orphaned son of his cousin, the Thomsonian herbalist Willard Richards, to be a doctor. Joseph S. Richards, already a druggist, also went to New York City, at Brigham's suggestion, where he entered Bellevue Hospital Medical College. He graduated in 1875 and returned to Utah to practice.[30] President Young also called women to be doctors. The first he called was Romania Bunnell Pratt, wife of Parley P. Pratt, Jr. After two tries, she graduated from the Woman's Medical College in Philadelphia in 1877 and returned to Utah to practice.[31] Another woman called by Brigham Young was Mrs. Ellis R. Shipp, who also graduated from Woman's Medical College. After returning to Utah, she began publishing Utah's first medical journal, the *Salt Lake Sanitarian* (188_90).[32] Another early Utah woman doctor was Martha Huges Paul, who graduated from the University of Michigan in 1880. Brigham also had a hand in her calling too.[33]

From all of this, the reader would be led to believe that President Young had finally decided in favor of medical science, and relaxed his former interest in the botanic way of healing. But here again the element of surprise enters in. For, during the same time that Brigham was calling these people to go back East to study medicine, he also called certain individuals to go back East and study herbal medicine at Thomsonian Schools of Botanic Science. One such person was Patriarch Elias H. Blackburn. On the completion of his course, he returned to Utah, and used his herbal knowledge in conjunction with the Priesthood, when called upon to heal the sick. He was successful in every case he treated. He would use a combination of herbal medicine, Priesthood power, and consecrated oil to work the needed cures desired. Sometimes he would just use the prayer of faith alone and the ordinance of administration. Other times he would just use herbs alone. But in this manner, and after this fashion did he work often among the sick. [34]

And during that interesting period of the 70s while these solicitations for skilled men and women of medical science were going out from the First Presidency at regular intervals, Brigham Young delivered several stern messages to the Latter-day Saints in the Tabernacle on Temple Square. As with previous sermons of an earlier vintage, they bespoke of a certain antagonism toward Gentile standards of medicine— the very same ones this man had urged a number of people to go East and study.

Sermon of September 16, 1871:

> *We do not know what to do for the sick, and if we send for a doctor he does not know any more than anybody else. No person knows what to do for the sick without revelation. Doctors, by their study of the science of anatomy, and by their experience, by feeling the pulse, and from other circumstances may be able to judge of many things, but they do not know the exact state of the stomach. And again, the operations of disease are alike on no two persons on the face of the earth, any more than the operation of the Spirit of God are alike on any two persons. There is as much variation in these respects as there is in the physiognomy of the human family; hence, when disease seizes our systems, we do not know what to do, and death often overcomes us, and we bury our friends. This is hard for us, but what of it. We will follow them; they will not come back to us.*[35]

Sermon delivered October 9, 1872:

> *Would you want doctors? Yes, to set bones. We should want a good surgeon for that, or to cut off a limb. Do you want doctors? For not much of anything else, let me tell you, only the traditions of the people lead them to think so, and here is A GROWING EVIL IN OUR MIDST. It will be so in a little time that not a woman in all Israel will dare to have a baby unless she can have a doctor by her.*[36] *I will tell you what to do, you ladies, when you find you are going to have an increase; go off into some country where you cannot call for a doctor, and see if you can keep it. I guess you will have it, and I guess it will be all right, too.*
>
> *Now the cry is, 'Send for a doctor.' If you have a pain in the head, 'Send for a doctor;' if you feel aches, 'I want a doctor;' 'my back aches, and I want a doctor.'*

The study and practice of anatomy and surgery are very good; they are mechanical, and are frequently needed. Do you not think it is necessary to give medicine sometimes? Yes, but I would rather have a wife of mine that knows what medicine to give me when I am sick, than all the professional doctors in the world. Now let me tell you about doctoring, because I am acquainted with it, and know just exactly what constitutes a good doctor in physic. It is that man or woman, who, by revelation, or we may call it intuitive inspiration, is capable of administering medicine to assist the human system when it is besieged by the enemy called Disease; but if they have not that manifestation, they had better let the sick person alone.

I will tell you why: I can see the faces of this congregation, but I do not see two alike; and if I could look into your nervous systems and behold the operations of disease, from the crowns of your heads to the soles of your feet, I should behold the same difference that I can see in your physiognomy—there would be no two precisely alike. Doctors make experiments, and if they find a medicine that will have the desired effect on one person, they set it down that it is good for everybody, but it is not so, for upon the second person that medicine is administered to, seemingly with the same disease, it might produce death. If you do not know this, you have not had the experience that I have.

I say that unless a man or woman who administers medicine to assist the human system to overcome disease understands, and has that intuitive knowledge, by the Spirit, that such an article is good for that individual at that very time, they had better let him alone. Let the sick do without eating; take a little something to cleanse the stomach, blood, bowels, and wait patiently, and let Nature have time to gain the advantage over the disease.

Suppose, for illustration, we draw a line through this congregation, and place those on this side where they cannot get a doctor, without it is a surgeon, for thirty or fifty years to come; and put the other side in a country full of doctors, and they think they ought to have them, and this side of the house that has no doctor will be able to buy the inheritance of those who have doctors, and overrun them, outreach them, and buy them up, and finally obliterate them, and they will be lost in the masses of those who have no doctors.

I want some say when they look at such things, but that is the fact. Ladies and gentlemen, you may take any country in the world, I do not care where you go, and if they do not employ doctors, you will find they will beat communities that employ them, all the time. Who is the real doctor? That man who knows by the Spirit of revelation what ails an individual and by that same Spirit knows what medicine to administer. That is the REAL doctor; the others are quacks.[37]

Excerpt from a sermon given August 31, 1875:

Instead of calling for a doctor, you should administer to them by the laying on of hands and anointing with oil, and give them mild food and herbs, and medicine you understand.[38]

Now, the preceding sermon of some length just given, deserves careful consideration. For, a close analysis of the same will reveal a clue as to the man's strange behavior in changing his stand so often.

First of all, he believed in doctors, but only to the extent of fractures, sprains, pulled ligaments, and such, with a surgeon for necessary amputation when they may occur. But in the third sentence is revealed by the Prophet of the Lord, the reason WHY he was inclined to sending several Latter-day Saints back East to learn the medicine of the world. It is BECAUSE A GOOD MAJORITY OF THE MORMON PEOPLE WANTED THESE SERVICES FOR THEMSELVES IN THE TERRITORY. And rather than suffer to see some corrupt Gentile practitioners come in and work their stuff upon the members of the Church, he felt that if they had to have doctors, they might as well have those of their own faith treat them. The territory had already been "blessed" with a few of those kind of the world, and he did not want any more if he could help it.

It's for the very same reason which he started up the Z.C.M.I. Organization. The Saints were patronizing the shops and stores of Gentile, "black-leg" (Heber C. Kimball's term) merchants and rather than see the wicked prosper, he felt to induce the Saints to shop at a Church-owned and managed department store, where at least the money would go toward building up the Kingdom of God instead of the Devil's. Preaching failed to discourage many from shopping outside of Mormon merchants and even threatened excomunications did not stop them; so he had to turn to the Z.C.M.I. plan as a last resort.

Thus, it was upon the same principles which he operated when he called certain men and women to go back East and enroll in schools of medicine. THE PEOPLE WANTED MEDICAL DOCTORS so Brigham felt to give them what they wanted; only he wanted them Mormon doctors, and not Gentile.

Brigham Young described the menace of Mormon dependence on medical doctors as A GROWING EVIL IN OUR MIDST! He even prophesied that the time would come when a Latter-day Saint mother would not dare have a child without the care and attention of a medical doctor attending her. Certainly, in our generation this has been fulfilled to the letter.

The only other item of great significance in his sermon is this: that a doctor, be it man or woman, should operate by revelation, both in diagnosing the sick and also in ministering medicine. That the true doctor, be it medical or herbal, is a revelator, or one who can receive revelation for himself in his specific practice. All others who do not, he labels as IMPOSTERS; or more bluntly, quacks. Certainly, if this principle of his was more strictly adhered to today by the men of medicine in the Mormon faith, there would be less of a chance of risk involved, both in the operating room as well as in the pharmacy, And there would not need to be the frequent explanation heard of the smiling doctor as he emerged from the operating room after surgery, proclaiming in joyful delight, "The operation was a success." And then mumbling at the bottom of his breath, "But the patient died." It is certainly something well-worth thinking about at least.

In the Fall of 1875, approximately two years before his death, he announced from the pulpit, a word of advice to the Saints at large; and that was to abstain from doctors, and resort to "mild foods, herbs, and medicine you understand." Thus, indicating he had not changed his mind nor entirely ruled out herbal medicine.

In the end however, the Hypocratic Oath[39] prevailed over his mortal remains, and when he died he was attended by three prominent medical doctors—his nephew Doctor Seymour B. Young, Doctors Joseph and Denton Benedict. How different from the days of Joseph and Hyrum, when the Prophet's own botanic physician, Dr. Levi Richards had custody of the bodies afterwards. And how different from when John Taylor was mortally wounded, and Dr. Levi Richards, the herbalist, attended him and nursed him back to health. Elder Taylor was not operated upon, but carried those bullets within his body for the rest of his life.

And yet, though these men of medicine administered such drugs as morphine[41] unto the dying Mormon leader to ease his terrible pain, somehow, in the end, his spirit prevailed over it all. For, the last three words which he uttered, before he expired his final breath, was the name of someone near and dear to him—not a close, personal friend—not a favorite wife or child—not even a fine physician—but rather instead, that of his beloved Prophet and Priesthood acquaintance, Joseph Smith. And, if Joseph had been there to receive him in the spirit, he would have understood that his brother in the flesh had tried throughout his entire life, to follow a course which would have been pleasing to God and the deceased Martyr as well. What finer tribute could "the greatest man next to Jesus Christ himself" have asked for, than that?

IN SUMMARY

1. Brigham Young counseled the men of the Mormon Battalion to let doctors and their medicine alone if they hoped to live.

2. The Men of the Mormon Battalion hated Dr. Sanderson with a passion.

3. Brigham Young was partial toward herbal medicine and medical science as well.

4. An herbal Council of Health in the Valley, superceded the Medical Association to follow some years later.

5. Too much dependence on medical doctors is "a growing evil in our midst."

6. Unless a doctor will allow himself to be guided by *revelation*, he has no business whatsoever practicing his skills upon the public.

CHAPTER EIGHT

THE END OF AN ERA

(The Passing of Herbal Medicine in the Mormon Church)

It seems that the great Mormon leader, Brigham Young, set a style and precedent for his successors to follow after him. In both sermons and actions the men of a later generation were to emulate him in what they had seen the Prophet of the Lord speak and do. For example, a typical sermon of Brigham's would usually go something like this:

LET THE DOCTORS ALONE

This counsel, emphatically given by our President in the Tabernacle on the 21st. inst., gave great satisfaction to every Saint present and we presume will be hailed with equal joy by every lover of truth whom it may reach. It might naturally be presumed that every member of the Church of Jesus Christ of L.D.S. was perfectly familiar with the revealed mode of curing disease and preserving health, but through the power of tradition the force of custom and habit, and on account of various weaknesses pertaining to the flesh, there has been quite a trusting to the fancied skill of man, quite a seeking unto the doctors who cannot save. And doctors, knowingly or ignorantly, often take credit to themselves for that which they do not effect, and thus foster a system which tends to weaken our faith, though it puts means easily into their possession. It does seem that the shallowest acquaintance with the different schools of medicine, with their diametrically opposite and conflicting theories and practice, with the known experimenting demonstrations with such various kinds of drugs upon so delicate and nicely arranged an organization as that of the human body, and all this in direct contrariety to the revealed will of Heaven, would serve to entirely prevent every Saint from seeking unto doctors, even though there were no commandments upon the subject. But unfortunately, such is not the fact; hence, the timely and very necessary testimony of our President upon the subject, and the most excellent counsel 'Let Doctors Alone,' which certainly should be the faith and practice of all who wish to live upon the earth until they have acceptably done the will of Him who gave them this, their probation.[1]

Herewith then, on the following pages, are some sermons and editorials reflecting the attitudes of the Church leadership in general during the turbulent 80s and the calming 90s. The reader will notice a distinct parallel between their messages, and the thoughts and sentiments of Brigham Young as contained in that synopsis just given before:

LIVING BENEATH OUR PRIVILEGES

When our friends are stricken down by sickness and disease or when our little ones are in the agonies of pain and death, there should be Elders in our midst who have educated themselves so thoroughly in developing the gifts of the Spirit within them, and in whom the Saints have such perfect confidence, that they would always be sought after instead of doctors. There are men among us who possess the gift of healing and might have great faith; but they do not exercise the gift; they do not live for it, and, therefore, do not have the power to use it so effectually as they might. There are men in this church who are as good in their hearts and feelings as men ever were, but lack faith and energy, and do not obtain really what it is their privilege to receive. If their faith, their energy, and determination were equal to their good feelings and desires, their honesty and goodness, they would indeed, by mighty men in Israel; and sickness and disease and the power of the evil one would flee before them as chaff before the wind. Yet, we say we are a good people, and that we are not only holding our own but making great advances in righteousness before God, and no doubt we are. But I wish to impress upon you, my brethren and sisters, that there are Elders among us endowed with spiritual gifts that may be brought into exercise through the aid of the Holy Ghost. The gifts of the Gospel must be cultivated by diligence and perseverance. The ancient prophets when desiring some peculiar blessing, or important knowledge, revelation or vision, would sometimes fast and pray for days and even weeks for that purpose...

—Apostle Lorenzo Snow, May 6th, 1882.[2]

TRUE FAITH AND WORKS

There is another tendency that is very noticeable among Latter-day Saints, and against which the voices of the servants of God should be lifted in continued protest, and that is the inclination that seems to be growing everywhere to resort to drugs and doctors when sickness enters the household, instead of having recourse to the means which God has commanded His people to use. The laying of hands for the healing of the sick is an ordinance of the Gospel. One of the signs which the Lord Jesus Himself promised His disciples in ancient days that should follow them that believed was 'they shall lay hands on the sick, and they shall recover.' In our day the promise has been renewed; and we claim it, for the Lord says:

'For I am God, and mine arm is not shortened; and I will show miracles, signs and wonders, unto those who believe on my name.

'And who do so shall ask it in my name in faith, they shall cast out devils; they shall heal the sick, they shall cause the blind to receive their sight, and the deaf to hear, and the dumb to speak, and the lame to walk.

'And the time speedily cometh, that great things are to be shown forth unto the children of men.'

Many, however, fail to avail themselves of these promises, and excuse themselves for doing so by saying that faith without works is dead. They seem to think that works consist in sending for a doctor and using what he may prescribe, having apparently more faith in man's skill than in God's power to heal through the ordinance which He has appointed. In saying this, we would not wish to convey any wrong idea. We believe it is the duty of those who have sick in their households to do all in their power for their comfort, to nurse them with the greatest possible care...the Lord says:

'And whosoever among you are sick, and have not faith to be healed, but believe, shall be nourished with all tenderness, with herbs and mild food, and that not by the hand of an enemy.

'And the Elders of the Church, two or more, shall be called, and shall pray for and lay their hands upon them in

my name; and if they die they shall die unto me, and if they live they shall live unto me...and again, it shall come to pass that he that hath faith in me to be healed, and is not appointed unto death, shall be healed.

'He who hath faith to see shall see; he who hath faith to leap shall leap; and they who have not faith to do these things, but believe in me, have power to become my sons; and inasmuch, as they break not my law, thou shall bear their infirmities.'

This is the Lord's teaching concerning the treatment of the sick who have not faith to be healed, and it should receive attention from the Saints. It is only reasonable to think that the Lord knows better that which is good for us than man does. His power to heal is without limit. He desires his children to exercise faith. By its exercise great blessings can be obtained. The more it is exercised and the oftener the results which are desired are obtained, the stronger does faith become.

Children who are taught by their parents to desire the laying on of hands by the Elders when they are sick, receive astonishing benefits therefrom, and their faith becomes exceedingly strong. But, if instead of teaching them that the Lord has placed the ordinance of laying on of hands for the healing of the sick in His Church, a doctor is immediately sent for when anything ails them, they gain confidence in the doctor and his prescriptions and lose faith in the ordinance.

How long would it take, if this tendency was allowed to grow among the Latter-day Saints, before faith in the ordinance of laying on of hands would die out? Little by little the practice of using drugs and resorting to men and women skilled in their use would grow among the people until those who had sick children or other relatives who did not send for a doctor when they were attacked with sickness, would be looked upon as heartless and cruel. Perhaps they would be taunted for not sending for some skilled person and perchance be condemned for trusting entirely to the ordinance of the Gospel and the proper nursing and kind attentions which every person who is sick should receive. There is great need of stirring up the Latter-day Saints upon this point. Faith should be encouraged. The people should be taught that great and mighty works can be accomplished by the exercise of faith. The sick have been healed, devils have been cast out, the *blind have been restored to sight by the exercise of faith. And this too, in our day, and in our Church, by the administration of God's servants in the way appointed. All these things can again be done, under the blessing of the Lord, where faith exists. It is this faith that we should seek to preserve and to promote in the breasts of our children and of all mankind.*

—*President George Q. Cannon,*
November 1st, 1893. [3]

SENDING FOR THE DOCTORS

... There will be but comparatively few of the human family that will attain to Celestial glory, because they will not listen to the Voice of God.

... If on the other hand, we desire a Celestial glory, and live for it, having a determination that with the help of God, we will be as our Savior was in the flesh—obedient, humble, meek and lowly, enduring all things for the glory that awaiteth us—then we shall attain to the fullness of that glory, and that reward will be bestowed upon us.... He wants the Latter-day Saints to attain to the highest glory.... And yet my brethren and sisters, when we examine ourselves, how far are we individually from coming up to it. Why, many of us cannot even obey the simple requirements embodied in the revelation concerning the Word of Wisdom. Many of us cannot rise high enough in our faith to pay an honest tithing. Many of us fail in living with that singleness of purpose and that unselfishness which the Gospel of the Lord Jesus Christ requires at our hands. Many of us have not faith enough even to send for the Elders of the Church when anyone of our family is sick; but the first thought is, 'go for a doctor'—as though the gift of healing had been lost in the Church. How many of you, my brethren and sisters, feel as if the gift of healing no longer exists in the Church of Christ, but that the doctor must be sent for, and drugs administered? And this among the Latter-day Saints, a people who profess what we do, and to whom such glorious promises have been made. Is not this true? It is so to one extent in Salt Lake City. I do not know how it is in this ward (Millcreek). I am scarcely ever called in to administer to a sick person without being told what the doctor is doing and what he says. To me IT IS AN EVIDENCE OF A WANT OF FAITH *in the ordinances of God's house and in His promises. To think of a people with the promises made to them that their sick shall be*

healed, if they only exercise faith, neglecting this, and treating it as though there was no certainty to be attached to it! It is the same in other directions. We fail to set a proper example before our young people. If I were to send for a doctor, what would be the effect upon my children? Why, they would say, 'That is the course my father took, and he is an Elder in the Church, and a man of experience; he sent for the doctors, and why should not I?' (Or) My mother was a good woman; but when one of the children was sick, she sent for a doctor; she did not trust to the ordinance alone; and shall we not send for a doctor. Must it be faith and no works? How often we hear this sort of reasoning? I believe in works, I believe in nursing, in taking care of the sick, and in doing all that is possible for them; but I also believe in the ordinances of the House of God. God has made precious promises to the Latter-day Saints concerning the health of their families, and I tell you in the presence of the Lord, that if the Latter-day Saints would observe the Word of Wisdom, there would be less of this disposition to send for doctors and more faith in the ordinance that the Lord has established... and let me tell you, there will be pestilence and there will be diseases; for the Lord has said that there should be an overwhelming scourge pass through the nations of the earth; and if the Latter-day Saints do not keep His counsel on this as well as other matters, how can they expect to enjoy immunity or receive deliverance?

I know that in talking this way I may grieve some persons, but shall we conceal the truth from the Latter-day Saints at this stage of our progress? Shall we say that the violations of the counsel of the Lord are right? ... He honors those who honor (the) Priesthood. No man can expect the blessings of God who does not honor the Priesthood of the Son of God.

...we must do as Jesus did from the beginning to the termination of His life, that is, do the Will of the Father as it is manifested to us, through the means He has provided....

—President George Q. Cannon
August 26th, 1894.4

INSTRUCTIONS TO THE SISTERS

At the late Relief Society Conference of the Utah Stake of Zion, held in Provo, Presidents John and Cluff both addressed the sisters, and among other important instructions, pleaded *earnestly with the mothers to cease building up the doctors and drug stores in our midst. Said Pres. Cluff: 'The doctors and druggist are getting enormously rich, and they are doing it at your expense. Our people are fattening them daily, and daily as a people are we drawing away from the principles of this part of our religion.' Pres. John followed in a powerful exhortation to the sisters to return to the early faith of the saints.... You have the plain, simple directions in the Doctrine and Covenants for your guidance, you have consecrated oil and can call in the power of the Priesthood, no matter how poor and destitute your circumstance may be, to assist you in this labor of love and healing, and yet the moment your children complain of a little illness you are off for the doctor...then (you) can feel you have got the skill of man on your side, while you leave the Priesthood to stand aside.[5]*

SENDING FOR DOCTORS SHOWS A LACK OF FAITH

...it is the doctors, however, and their erroneous practice that I desire more especially to write at present. The time was in this territory when physicians numbered but few and the families were limited wherein their services were required. At present, conditions are changed, and nearly every family residing in the neighborhood of a doctor are visited to a greater or lesser extent by him. The general experience is similar to that of a prominent man in one of our stakes as expressed to us recently: 'A short time ago we had no physicians in our stake and it was rarely that we felt the lack of one but since one located among us, sickness has increased so rapidly that we can now keep no such professionals going night and day to answer calls.'

If it is true that the hosts of doctors now in our midst find renumerative practice, then there must be some censure, due to the Saints for a disregard of the Lord's counsel. For there certainly has been an increase of disease and a consequent greater demand for medical services all out of proportion to the increase of population.

I have no doubt that we should very soon become a healthy and strong people if we would strictly follow the suggestions contained in the Word of Wisdom and the ordinary rules of health which common sense suggests; and then exercise faith in the ordinances of the gospel for the benefit of the afflicted, instead of sending for a doctor the moment we feel indisposed. THIS LATTER COURSE SHOWS A LACK OF FAITH. But unbe-

lief is natural where disobedience has been practiced.... It is a shame to us as a people that we neglect, as many of us do, the gifts of healing and the gift to be healed which the Lord has so mercifully given us. It is a disgrace that many possessing a mere smattering of medical knowledge can speedily obtain a practice netting annually thousands of dollars, while the great Giver of life, who knows how to provide every organ of the body is unsought in the hour of sickness. It is a standing reproach to us, we still place more reliance on the skill and knowledge of man, than on the power of God.

—Apostle Abraham H. Cannon[6]

HEALING BY FAITH

The custom of appealing to physicians for medical assistance in all cases of sickness has become as prevalent even among the L.D.S., that faith in the healing of the sick has been measurably relegated to the rear. It is true, we still send for the Elders, but the physician is, or will be, in the house as well, and we are apt to rely more upon his skill than upon the administration of the Priesthood. While if there is a return of health, we are pretty sure to give the credit to the physician.

This people are not narrow in their views on the subject of physicians, but we must sound a warning cry in the ears of the women of the Relief Society, that they fail not in their duty to teach lessons of faith in God and in the laying on of hands for the healing of the sick, to their families.

In the rise of this church, faith was the one and only recourse in all cases of sickness and disease. Simple remedies were administered and were perhaps a part of the household equipment. But the bottle of consecrated oil occupied the most prominent place in the sick rooms of the Latter-day Saints. The pages of the old Millennial Star teemed with the cases of miraculous healings under the hands of the Elders. Who is there that has not seen the wonderful healing made manifest among this people from time to time? Is there any lack of power in the Priesthood? On the contrary, there has probably never been more power and efficacy in the united ranks of the priesthood than at the present time. What, then, may be the difference? It is an entirely individual trouble. You and I, dear sister, may be at fault. The moment we are sick, do we take a remedy or hunt up a physician? And if we hear of a neighbor who has been taken ill, is our first question, who is the doctor, or what does the doctor say? Too much of our time in social affairs is spent in discussing medical problems and medical treatment. The children hear all this and consequently when they are sick their first thought is not to inquire for a spoonful of consecrated oil, but to lean upon the doctor and his advice.

If we are to retain the established principle of faith for the healing of the sick, we must work at it as we would at any other principle or doctrine which we wish to make a part of our lives. Whenever the need arises with ourselves, or with our dear ones, then call in the Elders, as we are told to do in the Scriptures, and if we are not healed on their first visit let us call them in again and yet again. The Lord will surely heal us if we surely call. We sometimes say we need a physician to tell us what ails us. The Lord is perfectly cognizant of our condition and he's able to heal one difficulty as another. I wish the sisters would read Alma's description of faith as given in Alma, chapter 32, verses 26-45, in this connection. This is the simplest and finest description of the manner in which we can acquire that wonderful gift of faith ever recorded in the Scriptures.

—Susy Young Gates, August, 1914.[7]

One Latter-day Saint sister living in those times, had this to say in connection with the above editorial just given, about the faith of certain medical doctors at the turn of the century in relation to the functions of the Priesthood:

I remember my grandfather, and the two brethren who came with him, administering to me, and how they, my parents and other relatives knelt around my bed and prayed that my life might be spared. When the doctors arrived, I recall that my folks decided to ask the Lord again for help in my behalf.

Someone said that if there was anyone in the room who did not feel like exercising faith for my recovery to please step out. BOTH DOCTORS LEFT THE ROOM. AFTER THE ADMINISTRATION, THE DOCTORS RETURNED AND THEY WERE AMAZED TO DISCOVER that I was no longer paralyzed and decided that an operation was not necessary. I was many weeks in bed, but slowly I improved. I had to learn to walk again. At the time, I was past six years of age. People living here, who knew of the circumstance, often speak of it and say, 'You are one person who has practically raised from the dead. It was a miracle.' Thus, my life was spared through Divine power. I have lived to become the mother of three sons and three daughters. I testify that this is the true Church, restored again in these the latter days, with all its promised powers, gifts and blessings.

—*Mrs. Sheila A. Carlile Winterton*[8]

Thus, we can see from the fore-going excerpts made of some classic sermons and editorials of the time, how certain perceptive individuals could see the trend toward doctors increasing among the Latter-day Saints, and made an effort to warn the people of God about this, and speak out against what they considered "a pernicious evil" growing in our midst. A member of the First Presidency, George Q. Cannon declared that there "is an inclination that seems to be growing everywhere to resort to drugs and doctors." And, he further remarked that "if this tendency was allowed to grow among the Latter-day Saints... faith in the laying on of hands would die out!" And also testifying to the people in his apostolic calling that resorting to such medical means was AN EVIDENCE OF A WANT OF FAITH on their part.

Other prominent figures in this crusade of warning against what they considered and felt to be "an evil in their midst," were stake presidents, such as those in the Utah Stake of Zion, who chided the sisters for placing more confidence in the skill of doctors and neglecting the Priesthood. Apostle Abraham H. Cannon raised his voice too against such methods adopted by the people of God, and told them that by resorting to the doctor every time they were sick "SHOWS A LACK OF FAITH!" And even the noted editor of the Relief Society Magazine, Susan Young Gates, felt inspired to warn the sisters that "if we are to retain the established principle of faith for the healing of the sick, we must work at it as we would at any other principle or doctrine which we wish to make a part of our lives."

However, such timely messages from inspired men and women of God seemed to go unheeded by the majority of the membership; for, we find that during the period from Brigham Young's death until the turn of the nineteenth century, the leadership of the Church, BECAUSE OF THE PEOPLE, were forced to resort to some of the same practices and policies which President Young had to adopt in the last seven years of his life.

Hence, as faith in the healing ordinance of the Priesthood gradually began to wane somewhat in Israel (as has just been proven from the preceding statements of quoted leaders then), the First Presidency of the Mormon Church became more and more responsible for such incidents of occurrence, as the following:

I had often accompanied Dr. Andreas Engberg on his professional visits, and this true friend of ours, and sincere well-wisher, had on various occasions, years before, suggested that I study medicine. And then on the road home one evening my wife inquired where Dr. Engberg and I went. I told her, and then she asked, 'Why don't you become a doctor?'

*So in the year of 1892, my wife and I decided that I study medicine, and I set about seeking the right kind of counsel as to the wisdom of such a step. Accordingly, I went to Salt Lake City to the office of the First Presidency, where I saw President Wilford Woodruff and George Q. Cannon, making known my intention and asking their advice whether or not to undertake the study of medicine. They replied that the Latter-day Saints should have professional men of their own faith and they unhesitatingly advised me to go right ahead and study medicine, if I possibly could reach it financially. They also advised me to come up to Salt Lake when I had completed all arrangements and before starting, when I would be set apart for the work contemplated. At the suggestion of Brother Andreas Engberg I decided to go to Cincinnati, Ohio, and enter the Eclectic Medical Institute, and I successfully passed the entrance examination and was allowed to matriculate. My satisfaction at my success so far can be imagined, when it is remembered that I had never yet seen the inside of a school, as a pupil. Before leaving for Ohio, I went to the First Presidency again where I was set apart as a missionary and to study medicine in the City of Cincinnati. Among other blessings pronounced by the servants of God on this occasion were the promises that I should learn fast, attain what I set out for, return in safety and be a comfort to the Latter-day Saints, who should have great confidence in me. I did complete my medical education...*9

Here then we have some of the first real evidences of "medical missionaries" to be found within the Mormon faith. However, their real origin began with President Brigham Young and was carried on by his successors after him. Other noteworthy accounts of this period worth mentioning are:

Father was suffering from arthritis and it was thought

wise to move to a warmer climate and the colonies of Northern Mexico seemed to offer the best situation, so, with neighbors, the family moved south by wagon train in the autumn of 1897. Through this move mother came into a situation that changed the course of her life. The colonies were without medical help. She began to sense that here, at least, was part of the call Aunt Zina Young had foretold in her blessing. As soon as she could make suitable arrangements, she went to El Paso hospitals for a refresher course in medical practitioner internship. Here she met the leading physicians and surgeons, became acquainted with hospital services offered and obtain a certificate to practice medicine under the laws of the State of Texas.[10]

The following summer Mrs. Young went East with her foster son, Willard Young. Her purpose was to gather the records of her relatives. Dr. Ellen B. Ferguson was one of the party on her way to New York to further pursue her medical studies. Prior to their departure the two ladies were set apart by the First Presidency of the Church to speak upon the principles of their faith as opportunity might be afforded. Mrs. Young was cordially received by her relatives and addressed, by invitation, Sabbath Schools and temperance meetings. She attended the Women's Congress at Buffalo, New York, but was refused five minutes in which to represent the women of Utah. She assisted, however, in organizing a Relief Society in that city. In 1893, at the Chicago World's Fair, she sat upon the platform as the representative of the women of Utah.[11]

But during these times, the old, natural ways of home remedy and practice had not been entirely forgotten:

In 1893 Zina D. Young, General President of the Relief Society of the Church of Jesus Christ of Latter-day Saints, accompanied President Wilford Woodruff in a canvass of the wards and stakes of the Upper Snake River Valley in Idaho, to invite women to attend a School of Medicine to be held in Salt Lake City under the direction of Dr. Margaret Curtis Shipp. President Woodruff emphasized that only women of courage, determination and abundant energy need apply, for they must be willing to endure hard work, long hours, and have the strength to battle the elements in their travel to the homes of those who needed aid. It was hoped that three women from each ward would qualify but only one from the Lyman Ward was in a position to go. Rachel B. Sutton wrote:

'My Mother, Sarah Susanna Blackburn Briggs, desired very much to take this course in medicine from Dr. Shipp....'

The following is taken from the diary of Mrs. Blackburn:

Dr. Shipp first gave us much advice on cleanliness, how to set bones, stop bleeding and to sew cuts. But the most important were the lessons given in midwifery and in the preparation and care of both mother and baby. At the conclusion of my training, I was promised by one of the Relief Society General Board members that if I would go to the Temple and ask the Lord to help me, I would be blessed. This promise was literally fulfilled, for though I delivered a few stillborn babies, I never lost a mother or baby in all my practice. When I was called to assist in childbirth I would drive my own horse and buggy to the home each day for ten days to bathe and care for the mother and baby. If the weather was bad, I would stay at the home for several days. I delivered several hundred babies over a period of twenty-seven years including three sets of twins.[12]

This was a kind of a carry-over from Brigham's day when midwives were to be considered as invaluable as a man's tool or horse would be:

Harriet Amanda Hoyt Bowers was born October 16 1850, in Salt Lake City Utah...

The Hoyts and Bowers followed their President's advice and settled in what was known as Winder later called Mt. Carmel where they were counseled to unite in an organization called the United Order. There were some who did not want to join, hence, people who wished to belong moved up the valley a few miles, and built a town they called Orderville. Each family had their own house and cared for their own families, but ate at the dining hall and had all things in common.

Harriet was called by President Brigham Young to be a midwife for the people of Orderville and was set apart by Erastus Snow. She received her training from Dr. Priddy Meeks and from him she learned the uses of herbs and roots. Her famed Liver Bitters and Cayenne Pills were used in most every home in Long Valley....[13]

But the lamentable passing of herbal medicine within the Mormon Church became significantly revealed with the establishment of the first medical hospital in that faith. A competent writer of Utah medical history observes the introduction of that system into Mormondom this way:

> *When any of the Saints became ill, they had in the absence of doctors, to rely on home remedies and the Lord. There were quite a number of midwives scattered through the settlements, who gave aid in cases other than childbirth. These women were self reliant and ingenious in treating the sick, and made up for their ignorance by their whole-hearted devotion to the nursing care of their patients.*

> *When home remedies and curatives to the afflicted were not enough, the Elders were called in. There were always several men in every community who held the Priesthood, which gave them the authority to administer to the ailing—that is, to apply the tenet of the Church that by anointing with oil, and the laying on of hands, with prayer, the sick could be healed! Under the circumstances, the Saints would have had nothing better, for it gave the afflicted hope and courage, faith in their eventual recovery and fortitude to endure their sufferings.*

> *Religious consolation to the sick and myriad is not peculiar to any one sect. Patients in well-equipped hospitals with everything that modern science can furnish for their recovery[1] sometimes lose their courage and morale in the face of impending danger. Their fears and forebodings may often be eased by a short visit from Rabbi, pastor, or priest. So it was entirely natural that the colonists in the colonies with no doctors or hospitals at their disposal should turn to the isolated Saints for Divine guidance and assurance of recovery.*

> *Before 1905, administration by the Priesthood took first place in the treatment of the sick. On January 9, 1902, the Dr. William A. Groves L.D.S. Hospital opened its doors for the reception of patients. That event was the first official acknowledgment by Church authorities that they were whole-heartedly behind scientific medicine and intended to give it moral and financial support. But the people were slow to accept and cooperate with the new movement. During the first few years of the hospital's activity, innumerable cases, particularly appendicitis, entered the hospital after several days of treatment by Priesthood administration. Most of their cases were in desperate condition, some too far gone for surgery. Nearly all of those operated on*

had peritonitis or abscesses and many of them died because of delay. Poor roads and horse transportation, doubtless played a part in the reluctance of patients to be taken to the hospital. As time passed, it improved, and scientific care was promptly sought. Administration was still widely practiced, but took a secondary place.

The Mormon people were not entirely dependent upon home remedies and religious administration. Scattered throughout the territory were several stalwart individuals, who dominated medical practice in their communities. These practitioners were herb doctors who had not studied medicine but had purchased Thomsonian certificates or graduated from the 'school of experience'...

On January 6th, 1905, there appeared in the Deseret News an editorial commenting on the fact that the. L.D.S. Hospital had been dedicated two days before.

The hospital is to be dedicated along the lines of 'Mormon' regulations...

The prayer of faith is efficacious in all forms of affliction. But all people have not faith to be healed, nor do all who have faith possess it in the same degree. Remedies are provided by the Great Physician or by Nature as some prefer to view them and we should not close our eyes to their virtues nor ignore the skill and learning of the trained doctor.

... It gives evidences that 'Mormon' enterprise is abreast of the times and that L.D.S. are ready to avail themselves of scientific knowledge and progress, and are not slow to move with the movement of modern thought and learning.[14]

Where the majority rules, even the Prophets sometime have to give way to the incessant demands of the people, and relinquish their firm stand on certain inevitable truths in order that the general membership be pacified. Such a condition existed more than once in ancient Israel. Under the able leadership of Moses, the children of God were given certain laws by which to be governed, and certain righteous ones called "Judges" to rule over them. But the main thing was that the people were FREE! They were not bound by an autocratic government, nor tied to a fetish system of things which might have been found in the known world then. They were under God's laws, God's prophets, God's judges, and

God's system of doing things.

However, when they looked around them and saw their Gentile neighbors on every side of them with a king here, and a ruler there, then they sought for the very same heathenish form of leadership that the others had. We find recorded in I Samuel 8:5 these words:

Then all the elders of Israel gathered themselves together and came to Samuel unto Ramah, and said unto him, Behold, thou art old, and thy sons walk not in thy ways; now make us a king to judge us like all the nations.

Being a Prophet who did not believe in compromise, Samuel was "displeased" with this sort of a request. He importuned the Lord in the matter several different times. The first time, God responded, He comforted Samuel by saying that they had not rejected Samuel but that they had REJECTED GOD HIMSELF! (see verse 7).

Samuel returned to the people, and under God's direction, sought to labor and reason with the people, in a plain manner of thinking. He rehearsed to them the matters of former kings of other nations with whom they had been acquainted. He pointed out the dangers of involuntary servitude, severe taxation, and compulsory rule, which existed with a king, if they allowed for one to be chosen in their midst. Despite this logical rationalization, the people wanted a king, nevertheless, and persisted in their demands upon Samuel. Wherefore, he returned to the Lord in the matter, and God sighed in exasperation at the obstinacies of His Children. He finally relinquished Himself in the matter, and told Samuel, "Hearken unto their voice, and make them a king!" (verse 22). Even He would not deprive them of their free agency, though it would mean the death and destruction of them anyway.

So Samuel chose Saul as the first king of Israel, and anybody acquainted with the Bible will soon learn how quickly Saul brought unhappiness, misery, and despair upon the people by his unrighteous conduct and wicked course of action. God saw it beforehand, but allowed it to happen anyway, because that's what THE PEOPLE WANTED!

Now then, we have the very same type of thing beginning in the Church toward the close of the last century. Because so much of the Gentile element and influence prevailed in the Territory, many of the people sought to adopt the ways and wiles of the world. This can certainly be evidenced in the fashions of the times. A young girl of that period, Violet Urie, recalls those times in these poignant words:

We kept our dresses long until some of the local women would go to Salt Lake City. When they returned we would learn that our dresses were too long for the city so that we would shorten our skirts a little when the word got around. We tried to dress accordingly to the city styles, and would be envious of the church leaders' daughters when they came to Cedar City in their high style clothes and their cut bangs and other new feminine styles.

When bang style came out, we were all anxious to try it. One older lady would preach against it every opportunity she had. She would talk in meeting and put the most gruesome story before us that we would be cursed with scabs and would become bald.

Mother would say, 'Now girls, if you are going to cut your hair a little, curl it and make it pretty. Tuck the ends under and then push it back away from your brow. Don't have your hair covering your brow.'

I wanted bangs in the worst way, so that I said to my sister, 'Florence, cut just a little here and there so I'll have some pretty curls.' Florence cut some short bangs across my forehead and oh, was I happy. I took my two long braids and wound them around and around so that only the little bangs showed underneath. Mother said, 'I'm glad you are happy; now you will sing better in the choir.' Mother was a diplomat. She never scolded or whipped us. She just needed to look at us, and we'd know what way we were to talk.

We were partakers of the world's wickedness, and the Lord forgive us for following styles, but many times we were just following the example of our church leaders' daughters. They would come to Cedar City so full of style that we would feel like we'd like to look just like them.

I remember President Taylor's daughter—coming to Cedar City. She had a dress that was twelve lengths at the bottom. My brother Will danced with her, and her dress filled almost the entire floor. She would hardly get so much material around her tiny waist. Her waist was so small, pulled in with heavy stays, that it looked as if a rounded forefinger and thumb would encircle it... [15]

113

And certainly the same held true with the Mormon people in other respects, such as in the field of medicine. The old pioneer way of steeping tea, or applying an herb poultice, or giving an herbal enema seemed now to become a piece of "old-fashioned nonsense" in the minds of many. When the younger generation coming up, saw the way the rest of the nation was taking care of its sick, through a system of clean-white hospitals, antiseptic doctors, and chemical medicine, then like Israel of old wanting a king, they earnestly sought for these same identical things to be within their faith and territory also. Hence, they prevailed upon their leaders to such an extent, that men like Brigham Young, George Q. Cannon, Wilford Woodruff, and Lorenzo Snow, who had personally known and been intimately acquainted with the Prophet Joseph Smith, now found themselves under the deplorable necessity of having to depart from some of the ways of their Revelator-friend, and adjust themselves to the times by adopting in certain measures of the world, which the people demanded of them. Joseph Smith hated doctors and had little use for Gentile medicine. This they knew and verily believed. But when the Saints at large began to patronize Gentile doctors and employ their services, the leading Brethren felt it would be better that the people go to Mormon doctors of their same faith. That is why they called some individuals to go back East and learn the medicine of the world; that thereby, the membership of the Church, who wanted these things, could have them. At last, the world which Brigham Young had sought to escape and leave, had finally arrived in the valleys of the mountains, and from there on into the twentieth century, Gentile medicine was here to stay!

A candid testimonial to the above assertion, is herewith provided by one who lived in those times, and saw the "age of compromise" slowly creep into the Mormon religion. Such a one, who witnessed these things for himself, was none other than James Henry Moyle, the father of the late President Henry D. Moyle, a counselor in the First Presidency of the Mormon Church, under the leadership of the deceased Prophet David O. McKay. The following is in Brother Moyle's own words:

Again fifty years ago, and for a long time afterwards, it was a rare and serious occasion when a doctor was called to serve the sick, unless a surgeon was needed to amputate or try to save a limb, or an injured member of the body. Such was the practice in my father's family and with practically all of our neighbors. The first thought in my mind, and in that of my devoted mother and our neighbors, was to follow the advice of James: 'If there are any sick among you, call the elders and let them anoint with oil, and the prayer of faith shall heal the sick.' (James 5:14)

When our neighborhood learned that the President of the Church and the chief officers of the Church had regularly attended physicians whose services were actively called into use even when the sickness was not serious, it was something of a shock. In Salt Lake City, the custom spread, especially as wealth increased, until now it is the rule rather than the exception. The money notwithstanding, it was a fact that remarkable cures were frequently if not commonly, effected by the administrations of the elders and the faith of the patient and his family, and with the aid of an uneducated, pioneer mother's remedies. In my very early life we neither knew of nor had heard of dangerous disease germs, and social diseases were intolerable and confined to the criminals and their unfortunate associations.

As a child, if I were sick and felt seriously ill, my first anxiety and request was that the elders of the Priesthood should be called to administer to me. My faith was implicit that I would be healed, and I was. Mother was a REAL pioneer, and she gave me tea, castor oil, herbs, and other home remedies and applied herbal applications for bruises, strains, and other injuries. If the trouble was obstinate, Daddy Bussel from across the street, an old English herbalist, was called. I never had a doctor until about sixteen or seventeen when it became necessary to amputate my left forefinger. Mother had thirteen children, which in those days was a common but crowning achievement among good Mormon women, but now shocking to many. I was the oldest. No doctor ever aided Mother at childbirth and such was the case with most neighbors unless something very serious developed. Mother never had any aid except from Sister Duncanson, an old Scotch neighbor who brought into the world all the babies in the neighborhood. There might have been an exception which I do not recall, but it would be only another less popular midwife. I do not think Mother remained inactive ever for more than two weeks. She invariably felt ready to resume her active duties in about a week. The midwife had difficulty in keeping her in bed over a week, if that long. She was unusually strong and healthy. I am sure her life would have been prolonged if she had not been so strenuous and prolific.[16]

It's much like the artificial turf they use today in some of the newer indoor stadiums and sports arenas. It costs more than the regular sod, but the upkeep is so much handier to deal with. You don't have to water it, or weed it, or mow it. It is neat, convenient and easy to take care of and maintain. There is not much fuss and bother to it.

Modern medicine is the same way. Drugs, while more expensive than herbal teas, generally do work faster in the system. The tiny timed-released capsules of "the Excedrin set" are truly most marvelous and amazing as well. "Shots," though they hurt, are quicker than herbal poultices, and certainly a lot less messy. Surgery is quick and painless, thanks to the "funny-gas" of modern anesthesiology. And modern medicine is quite adept at "casting" an individual with a fracture or sprain, in a supporting role of crutches. In all, the benefits to be derived from medical science are as numerous and varied as what Social Security may have to offer.

With the advent of medical science into the Mormon religion, the last breaths and gasps of a dying practice (botanic medicine) were to be heard in the wheezing coughs and choking closes of the nineteenth century. The *real* grass, Nature's stuff, had simply been replaced with an artificial turf. But was the latter any better?

IN SUMMARY

1. The prophet Joseph Smith's herbal medicine went out of the Mormon Church, when the gentile medical science of the world came in!

CHAPTER NINE

ARE WE A PECULIAR PEOPLE?

(The Place of Herbal Medicine in Mormonism Today)

With the evolution of modern medicine, one would naturally be inclined to ask, "Have we been able to retain our identity as a peculiar people?" In the light of recent changes made down through the years in the second century of Mormonism, some scholars have been in a quandary as to how they should answer this. Two such men, both distinguished professors of history at Brigham Young University, made this interesting observation in their fine treatise "Mormonism In the Twentieth Century:"

> *After Reed Smoot was finally given his Senate seat in 1907,* MORMONISM DECLINED AS A CONTROVERSIAL ISSUE....
>
> *During the decade beginning in 1930, the centennial year of Mormonism, two new features were seen in the popular image which have characterized it ever since. Although the long-range trend had been toward a more favorable image, it was not until these years that it crossed the line from a predominantly negative to a more positive character. The second new feature was a strong interest in the program of the Mormon Church rather than in its theology. This change reflected a general shift seen in twentieth century American religion—interest in the 'social gospel' and its program for social salvation rather than in traditional emphasis on personal salvation through the atonement of Jesus Christ.*[1]

Thomsonian medicine was a controversial innovation into the field of hygenic science. When the man Thomson developed his system, he incurred much prejudice and trouble from the biased sector of American Society, chiefly the medical profession is existence then. As has been already mentioned in a quote from Priddy Meeks in the chapter touching on this system, Thomson's theories and practice rivaled the Gospel of

117

Jesus Christ which Joseph Smith introduced. Both had to suffer tremendously for the things in which they believed most strongly, and espoused most sincerely.

The very fact that the Prophet himself embraced this concept of new thinking, and made it a part of his religion while he was alive, in and of itself, made the new theology of Mormonism, a strange and unusual faith to the outside world not acquainted with it and its adherers—a "peculiar people." Most all Christian sects of the time accepted whatever there might have been of medical science as a standard norm of procedure to follow when sick. But the Mormons were different. They had "inspired Men of God" telling them to use herbs, trust in Almighty power, and secure the Priesthood whenever they were ill or had disease in their midst.

In fact, one of the charges hurled against the Latter-day Saints by their Gentile enemies, in Missouri, was this:

> *They still persist in their power to work miracles. They say they have often seen them done; the sick are healed through herbs and faith, the lame walk, devils are cast out; and these assertions are made by men heretofore considered rational men and men of truth...* [2]

Thus, the Mormon people were pegged from the very beginning as being "peculiar," "strange," "odd," "weird," and all other sorts of unexplainable adjectives. But the fact remains, that when the "nonsense" (as some think it to be) of herbal medicine left the Mormon Church, and its leaders no longer practiced it themselves, nor openly advocated it, then no longer were we "peculiar" to the rest of the world in this respect. For we now have their medicine and large, fine general hospitals the same as they do, and competent men of skill to practice therein, so how are we really any different from the rest of the Gentiles?

Perhaps, one significant thing which has happened of late has been the release of all Church-owned hospitals from the system of Mormonism altogether. And this inspiring piece of action done by a modern-day Prophet, who had the foresight and thought to declare that "we were in the business to preach the Gospel, not the hospital business." His prompt decisions, for whatever reasons upon which they were based, certainly deserve some distinguished note of laudable merit. A modern Prophet working under modern revelation, the same as his predecessors did under former revelation, to make the Latter-day Saints "a peculiar people" as we should be in the first place. And his wonderful efforts in the tremendous missionary program of the Church is another beautiful example of our "peculiarity." For what system of religion upon the face of the earth, or what faith in the land is there, that can rival the kind of proselyting action which the Mormon Church is now noted to have? Again, "a peculiarity" of "a peculiar people."

But, there have been some writers in modern times, friendly to the Mormon cause, who, nevertheless, have observed a waning of the "peculiarity" about which we are now speaking. One such man was Hector Lee, who conducted an extensive search throughout the Church to find material among the Mormons upon the subject of The Three Nephites. He interviewed hundreds of people, read countless diaries and journals, and, in general, did a rather thorough piece of work altogether. From all of these earnest efforts, he happened to make this revealing discovery:

> *Casting out devils, having visions, receiving revelations, talking in tongues, and similar physic phenomea are decreasing because the Church has either openly discouraged them or has avoided encouraging them, and because the appeal of the Church is shifting from the emotional (characteristic of the 1830s and 1840s)[3] to the rational, scientific, social and cultural.*

Another authority who noticed this "shifting from the emotional to the rational, scientific, social and cultural" in Mormon doctrine and theology was the noted sociologist Nels Anderson, who attributed this rather surprising change to the phenomena of education. In his book, Desert Saints, he makes the following analysis:

> *On the other hand, this striving for knowledge, this drive for education to promote the Kingdom of God, was an effort to conserve in the Mormon group the cultural values developed on the frontier. On the other hand, the education fetish has resulted in reversing intellectually all the old processes of pioneer insularism. It has forced the Mormons to turn around. It used to be a sin to 'approximate after the things of the world.' That was the justification for the Deseret alphabet—to shut out the intellectual influences of the Gentiles. There was no concern about approval of outsiders; in fact, disapproval was a compliment.*

> *This is no longer true, Zion was turned from insularism to identification—a process which has been speeded by the modern striving for the knowledge that comes in books, an interest that never greatly concerned the pioneers. There is a*

practical reason for this reversal. The urge for identification is more a matter of expediency than is generally realized even by the Mormons and is as much a matter of expediency as was the pioneer urge for isolation...

Perhaps this is the long-predicted expansion of Zion to the world, another kind of missionary movement. Certainly it is not a military, old-fashioned evangelical approach to the outside. On the contrary, the Mormons are now themselves on the other side. They are straining to adapt themselves. They have succeeded so well that their name is no longer anathema. Preachers no longer sermonize about the menace of Mormonism. Is this dilution process thinning out the old distinctiveness? Will Mormonism spread and adapt until it loses its identity. This has not happened YET![4]

When Mr. Anderson made this observation in the years of 1940-42, he was not aware what an additional 33 to 35 years would do to Mormonism. Mr. Anderson's thoughts, carefully gleaned from a long period of patient study, might, perhaps, be best summed up in these few words of the Savior, as recorded in the Gospel of John 15:18-19:

If the world hate you, ye know that it hated me before it hated you.

If ye were of the world, the world would love his own; but because ye are not of the world, but I have chosen you out of the world, therefore the world hateth you.

This turning from pioneer "insularism to identification" through "the modern striving for knowledge" (or education) has placed the Latter-day Saints in a very unique position, as being one of the fastest growing, most successful religious organizations upon the face of the earth. The "world-wide" Church of Jesus Christ of Latter-day Saints, in fact, has become one of the most popular institutions in existence today.

When two of the major television networks in this country (NBC and CBS) devote a half-an-hour of prime-time programming upon the subject of Mormonism, and when one of the most respected and prominent magazines in the world (The National Geographic) provides over a dozen pages about the Utah-based faith, then surely that is evidence enough to indicate we are a popular people with the world in general. Or, to requote MORMONISM IN THE TWENTIETH CENTURY, "Mormonism (has) declined as a controversial issue..." Since 1930 "new features were seen in the popular image which have characterized it ever since."

And yet, the question still remains to some extent, has all of this recognition, positive-image, and popularity caused us to lose our *original* identity as a peculiar people? How about the "peculiarity" those Gentile Missourians noticed about us—"they say...the sick are healed through herbs and faith ...."—Could this have been lost to some extent when Mormonism embraced the Gentile medical science of the world?

These questions are raised in earnestness because they have a direct bearing upon this whole work. Certainly, herbal medicine and botanic physicians today, meet with a frown of disgust and wince of chagrin to many who believe in the other. You mention the word "nature doctor," if you're telling someone about your visit to a local practitioner for some type of a complaint you're suffering from, and immediately the party to whom you're conferring such news, looks at you as if you are abnormal.

In part, their doubt and disbelief can be understood in the light of recent events the past few years. Of a truth, there have been a number of slick individuals who have operated out of back rooms with drawn window shades, in a variety of methods and techniques that are simply ridiculous to even the average-minded person. Machines that hum, lights that blink, and horns that sound, are no guarantee that cancer will be eliminated, nor brass, copper, and other attractive metal objects of dreamt-up names as a means of remedying other specific types of diseases. There is a point where the line has to be drawn, and this is it.

Certainly the medical profession in the State of Utah deserves a fine hand of commendation for their determined crusade against such shysters and rogues who prey upon the innocent and unsuspecting with gadgets and gimcrackery that even the old eccentric toy-maker Rube Goldberg would have nothing to do with. But has not that well-intentioned zeal gone just a bit far, when it includes honorable men of respected standing in the community? Is it right to spread the flame of determination upon trained specialists in the herbal and botanic sciences, who are licensed and qualified practitioners in their field as much as the medical men are in theirs? Isn't this depriving a man of his free agency if he is operating within the bounds and limits of proper authority, and conducting his practice in such a noble manner as would merit a nod from the deceased Prophet, Joseph Smith himself? Is it justice to defame a man because he prescribes herbs and other natural remedies to his patients instead of drugs and apothecary medicine? Is this the right way?

Now, there are in the State of Utah a class of men who are registered and licensed botanic physicians. They are called "Nature Doctors" by them who employ their services. These men base their practice upon more than just the Thomsonian cure of treatment. In fact, whereas lobelia used to be the "cornerstone of herbal faith" then, the plant, golden seal, has taken its place; and is now considered by some, to be "the thing" for nearly everything. Even herbal medicine has made significant strides since the days of Mr. Thomson!

Many of these men are also qualified medical doctors, and can give X-rays, immunizations, and regular medicine just as any ordinary M.D. can. They have been trained in this, and their diagnosis of something can be considered just as reliable as the physician's can be. But they have had to pay a price and, sometimes, bear a grudge from those in standard medical practice, when entering business for themselves. Like Mr. Thomson, they have found the way to the top not always an easy one to reach.

And then there have been those less fortunate than these, who because of limited finances could not afford the schooling these other men had, or simply did not want to take the regular courses in order to qualify for a medical license with which to operate. These unlucky fellows have been arrested, tried, convicted, and in some cases, even sentenced to the state prison for the help they were attempting to administer to people. We do not mean the charlatans, but those who believed in herbs alone, and sought to use them without the aid of further medicine. Names could be mentioned, but this is not a martyr-sheet for roll call. It is merely a page of condensed facts which now exist in the heart of Mormondom, and are there with the counterparts in modern medicine.

But the question still remains, "Are we a peculiar people?" Well, perhaps, the presence of these men in a state dominated by the medical profession helps, somewhat, to lessen the image that we are an ordinary people, and at least stimulates the peculiarity factor to a small measure. However, what can be said about the Mormon people themselves? Are they "peculiar" anymore, or has Gentile medicine so affected them that they cannot be influenced anymore toward the natural method of cure?

Part of the answer may lie in this: Despite the radical changes within Mormonism after the turn of the century, yet there were still a few people among the Latter-day Saints who either believed in the use of herbs for sickness, or recommended their virtues to others. One such illustration may serve the point just given, rather well. In 1905, an old Mormon patriarch suggested the use of tobacco to an ailing young man of his faith, who could not obtain relief from anything else, medicine included. The account goes like this:

> David had saved a little of the money from the sale of our Mt. Pleasant home, also earning some money from herding sheep awhile. We bought the Decker home where Victoria and John lived for awhile. David got some work at Pinedale. Later he began with convulsions like Georgie had done. We later realized that when they both would lie upon their stomachs and drink from the edge of the creek where various creatures were, as some other boys also used to do; and, at the same time drank from the edge of the creek, drank eggs or tiny young ones of the 'nemotode' worm or snake. Georgie, while dying, declared there was a 'snake in his belly;' also, the same symptoms proved they both suffered from the same evil.

> I am very sorry now that we didn't have Georgie's entrails opened; then we could have known better how to deal with the evil creature in David. It would crawl up his chest at times until he could hardly breathe. We thought it was worms. We hadn't means to go to the doctor so far away. Besides, there didn't seem to be doctors then, especially in Arizona, who would understand about such creatures in the system. We finally decided it wasn't worms because different kinds of worm medicine did no good.

> Then, Patriarch John Riedhead of Woodruff, where Victoria lived, told me when I went down there, to have David try chewing tobacco and swallowing the juice, which would kill a snake and should kill anything else. Although David shrank at the thought of using tobacco, he was driven to try it; but he didn't get relieved then, of the misery which came at intervals...

> Finally, David's condition got so bad (the Spring of 1921), that he got to swallowing tobacco juice as Brother Reidhead advised; also used even very strong medicines. Those he took would only stun the creature inside of him for awhile; then it would go to work again. Besides the tobacco juice, he took rather loose food such as rice, soaked bread, etc., so the tobacco juice could mix with it in his stomach and the worm would have no place, but to be covered with the juice. The last three days of that treatment, the creature flopped about and made him awful sick—almost put him in serious convulsions, although he had had convulsions for some time. He kept taking the juice when he

felt the creature coming up into his throat; again, it would be stunned. It was struggling hard before it was killed.

Finally, it stopped moving at all, but David didn't know it was dead, so he kept taking the juice. The creature was so large that I knew if it was dead I must get him some medicine to take it away. I had a time getting across the wash that was full of deep muddy water on my four mile trip to Taylor. I took off my shoes and stockings and waded across. I got him some native herb tablets, but after he took them they heated him so that he took to shaking all over his body. His nerves were terribly bad. I got so worried about him that I went and talked with nurses I knew. Someone said to give him salts. I decided if they wouldn't help him, I would have to get a doctor. But we didn't have money. Joseph had been in France at war (WWII), but I didn't get all the checks that should have come. The doctor lived 40 miles from us and I didn't know hardly what to do. I gave David the salts and it was 3 weeks after he began to take the extra strong tobacco juice that he got rid of the creature.

It had been dead about two weeks and was almost to pieces; but it was an awful thing. It was over a foot long. It had burst but looked like it had been about as big around as my finger. It had a lot of joints about one-third of an inch long. It was whitish—that is, looking like an angleworm not filled with mud. It's head was peculiar, something like a snake's head, but didn't have bones or teeth. Someone told me that if it had teeth it would have killed David but it just sucked its food. Each one of those joints was pointed on the under side. It must have had four legs, but we saw only three. They had little claws and it was those that helped to hurt David at times. They were about as big around as a wheat straw and were half an inch to an inch long and quite near its head. Some folks thought it was a tape worm, but we saw pictures afterwards in a paper that described and showed pictures of 'nemitode' worms, which were a species of a snake.

David got much better after he got rid of the creature, although it had made his stomach bad. He had also suffered much with piles, but now he got them better. He had been so pale and weak, but he got strong; even grew in size and went out at quite heavy work.

After David got rid of that snake he decided to burn his

tobacco. I told him he may need it as it may be hard to quit, but he burned it anyway. Then I had to buy more, as he got into a terrible nervous condition before he got well. But he finally got the habit conquered, too. 5

And even one of the General Authorities, Apostle John A. Widstoe, believed in living naturally. Now, as to whether or not he ever used herbs directly for sickness, cannot be said as that fact is not definitely known. But this much can be authenticated from his daughter, Ann Wallis:

My father never seen a medical doctor in his life. He never went to a dentist. And, he never was sick one day, that I know of. For the last twenty years of his life, he ate no meat, but confined his diet strictly to vegetables, fresh fruit, nuts, berries, and such as that. He lived to be 80 years old, and always seemed to have pep and energy about him. I never knew him to use any bleached flour, refined sugar, or processed foods of that type. Mother always cooked with wholesome ingredients—i.e., stone-ground whole wheat flour, honey, etc., etc. 6

Thus, with these two isolated incidents, we can see that to some small degree, the practice of herbal medicine and herbal dieting persisted after the nineteenth among those few who believed in such things. To this extent then, was the "peculiarity" of the Mormon people preserved, and its original identity with the Prophet Joseph in this regard, not lost entirely. And today, among a rather modest number, this belief and practice still prevails. It is unfortunate, however, that in many cases, where you might find a "health-food addict," you are also liable to find an individual with some theological or political hang-up besides. It seems that these sorry people have become fanatics in something which should be followed just as naturally as you would a path along which to walk. Rather instead, they seek to push the "natural way of health" to such a bitter extreme, that they make for themselves enemies, as well as to give other earnest seekers a bad name and deplorable reputation, when connected with the health-food line. And a few have even pressed their luck so far as to get excommunicated from the Mormon Church, because of their radical differences and non-conformity doctrines, which they stress so urgently as a matter of "life and death salvation" to others.

The author is here treating a type of "peculiarity" which is both obnoxious and bad, to medical Saint and herbal Saint alike. But, there are a remnant remaining, in hither unknown parts of the Church, who believe in and advocate the Prophet Joseph Smith's teaching in regards to herbal

medicine and practice it for themselves, their families, and close relations. These individuals do not belong to any "off-shoot" group, or
"pseudo" cult of fantastic imaginations. They are men and women like
ourselves—humble followers of Christ, who sustain the living Prophet of
God, and are active members of the Church of Jesus Christ of Latter-day
Saints.

It is these with whom the author refers to in good, honorable
intentions. Not so much for what they believe in and advocate, but rather
for their courage in daring to be DIFFERENT! Not the kind of "different"
that gets you in trouble with church authorities, but the kind of
"different," which is a free and easy style of simple "peculiarity." Not the
kind that's forced and preached in radical tones of apostate loudness; but
rather that which is a part of their normal, everyday lives, lived out in
submission, meekness and humility; walking obediently in all of the right
paths which God's living Prophets today prescribe! And yet, somehow,
managing to cling to the past and retain the identical ways of faith and
healing, which Brother Joseph himself maintained and kept throughout
his life. Or, in other words, the type of living pattern which John A.
Widstoe himself sought to establish; the kind that allows you to do your
"thing," and someone else to do his "thing."

But one last type of "peculiarity" must be raised before we close
this chapter and end our discussion. And that has to do with FAITH in the
healing ordinances of the Gospel. If the reader will kindly recall, there
have been in the last two chapters numerous statements by Brigham
Young, George Q. Cannon, Apostle Abraham H. Cannon, and Susan
Young Gates in regards to the administration of the sick. And be aware to
please remember that they all were rather unanimous in this one
message: FREQUENT RELIANCE UPON MEDICAL DOCTORS
SHOWED A LACK OF FAITH IN GOD! In fact, Susan Young Gates
herself said that "If we are to retain the established principle of faith for
the healing of the sick, we must work at it as we would any other principle
or doctrine which we wish to make a part of our lives." And the two Presidents John and Cluff, stated to the sisters in the Relief Society
Conference of the Utah Stake of Zion: "...the moment your children
complain of a little illness you are off for the doctor...then (you) can feel
you have got the skill of man on your side, while you leave the Priesthood
to stand aside." And, of course, Apostle Abraham H. Cannon eloquently
versed it in this manner when he said: "...sending for a doctor...SHOWS
A LACK OF FAITH!"

One of the "peculiarities of faith" which Jesus said should accompany His disciples who believed in Him, and *had confidence* in His power

and those of His Servants was this:

> *And these signs shall follow them that believe; in my name shall they cast out devils; they shall speak with new tongues; they shall take up serpents; and if they drink any deadly thing, it shall not hurt them;* THEY SHALL LAY HANDS ON THE SICK, AND THEY SHALL RECOVER! 7

Nowhere can a person read into this the interpretation of an inspired physician whose hands are directed by God in order that life might be preserved. Some would like to think it is this way; and still, many others tend to believe that "doctors are God's inspired servants and He works through them." Well, this may be the case sometimes; the author will not dispute that. But here Christ is talking about a *specific* type of a servant—not a skilled, medical practitioner, but rather a *Priesthood holder skilled in faith*! And when that certain bearer lays his hands upon the sick, THEY SHALL RECOVER! Or, in other words, the Savior is making a plain allowance for those who are to heal when faith and belief are present. When they are not, then it must be presumed he has made other provisions with which we are all very well acquainted.

It seems the early period of the Church enjoyed a remarkable out-pouring of the gifts and graces of God; to such an extent in fact, that one Elder in remarking upon such matters as visions, prophecies, tongues, etc. in his daily journal, was led to simply write on one occasion: "Nothing much out of the ordinary today...just the usual tongues, visions, etc...."8 However, we find in our searching, that a different attitude had been assumed about these things and the frequency with which they had appeared in the Church later on in another era.

Violet Ure was born August 10th, 1873. She wrote a short autobiography about herself when she was 87 years old, and resided at Cedar City, Utah. The original is on microfilm at the Church Historian's Office in Salt Lake. The author made this excerpt from her copious notes in the Archives:

> *...It seems the best time of my life was hearing people speak in their broken English. We would go to Fast Meetings and hear the brethren speak in their native tongues, in broken English, and even 'in tongues.' I look back on those days as being very precious to me,* FOR THE GIFTS OF THE GOSPEL WERE SCARCE IN THEM DAYS. *There were no doubts nor misgivings for those men, and they passed their strength to those who listened. With great power they would declare the gospel to be*

true.

Now, Sister Ure had written the above sometime in 1960. According to her age and the time she was born, it is interesting to note her significant statement that "THE GIFTS OF THE GOSPEL WERE SCARCE IN THEM DAYS." If this was true, and considered in the light of statements from men like George Q. Cannon and Abraham H. Cannon, together with the brief remarks of Susan Young Gates, about "a waning of faith" or "lack of faith" in demonstration of trust with medical aid, is it improper to ask JUST WHAT SORT OF A SPIRITUAL HERITAGE DID OUR ANCESTORS LEAVE US AFTER 1900?

Perhaps that can best be answered by Emily Dow Partridge Young, a daughter of the first Presiding Bishop of the Church, Edward Partridge, and a later wife of Brigham Young. As early as 1880, when the momentum of our present-day results bequeathed to us by our pioneer forefathers then, had begun to gather some acceleration toward the Gentile influences of the outside world, this noble woman heroically recorded:

> *... I speak of the gift of healing by the laying on of hands. But do we enjoy that blessing to the extent that we might.... We suffer with sickness year after year and children die.... Who is responsible for this state of things? Is it not those who are entrusted with the priesthood; holding the power and authority to rebuke the Destroyer? Are they not responsible in a great measure for the lack of faith among the people? Mothers having sick children send for the Elders according to the revelation; they come from their work feeling in a very great hurry. They cannot take time to bow down before the Lord and dedicate themselves, then administer and act concerned to His Glory, but go through the ceremony in a hurried manner, their minds filled with the cares of business. They think not of the result of their administration; but leave the patient or friends to exercise faith if they can under the circumstances. Who can wonder that distrust creeps into the minds of the people, and they send for a doctor rather than trust in an Elder when sickness is raging...*

> *We lose confidence in the Priesthood. J.S. and his brethren obtained blessings through much prayer. If there were two or three together, they would pray in turns and if they did not prevail at first, they would pray again and again until the Lord would grant them their desires. I have known Elders to lay on hands with no effect at first; but after the second or third*

*time, the patient was healed. Now, if it can be done once it can be done again and again.... I have been administered to repeatedly, without the desired effect; and I long to see the day when the Spirit and Power of healing will attend the administrators...*9

To dispute the facts, and close our eyes to the obvious, is certainly not a very intelligent sign of good common sense, is it? Therefore, what do we have to consider in the light of this recent evidence? Who can dare gainsay the difference about these matters? We leave the reader to be the sensible judge of what already seems to be so apparent.

The "peculiarity" of the Mormon style today appears more as an individual trait of a single character here and there, rather than as an aggregate measure of the entire sum quality everywhere. And it is this personal "peculiarity," unrelated to the masses in general, which helps to still identify Mormonism with some of the old teachings in Brother Joseph's day.

A classic example of this "individual peculiarity" to which we are referring, may be found in the life of Daniel and his friends, as related in the Good Book. We read as follows, in Daniel 1:1-20, of the *Inspired Version*:

In the third year of the reign of Jehoiakim king of Judah came Nebuchadnezzar king of Babylon into Jerusalem, and besieged it.

And the Lord gave Jehoiakim king of Judah into his hand, with part of the vessels of the house of God; which he carried into the land of Shinar to the house of his god; and he brought the vessels into the treasure house of his god.

And the kind spake unto Ashpenaz the master of his eunuchs, that he should bring certain of the children of Israel, and of the king's seed, and of the prince's;

Children in whom was no blemish, but well favored, and skillful in all wisdom, and cunning in knowledge, and understanding science, and such as had ability in them to stand in the king's palace, and whom they might teach the learning and the tongue of the Chaldeans.

And the king appointed them a daily provision of the king's meat, and of the wine which he drank; so nourishing them three years, that at the end thereof they might stand before the king.

Now among these were of the children of Judah, Daniel, Hananiah, Mishael, and Azariah;

Unto whom the prince of the eunuchs gave names; for he gave unto Daniel the name of Belteshazzar; and to Hananiah, of Shadrach; and to Mishael, of Meshach; and to Azariah, of Abed-nego.

But Daniel purposed in his heart that he would not defile himself with the portion of the king's meat, nor with the wine which he drank; therefore he requested of the prince of the eunuchs that he might not defile himself.

Now God had brought Daniel into favor and tender love with the prince of the eunuchs.

And the prince of the eunuchs said unto Daniel, I fear my lord the king, who hath appointed your meat and your drink, for why should he see your faces worse liking than the children which are of your sort? Then shall ye make me endanger my head to the king.

Then said Daniel to Melzar, whom the prince of the eunuchs had set over Daniel, Hananiah, Mishael, and Azariah;

Prove thy servants, I beseech thee, ten days; and let them give us pulse to eat, and water to drink.

Then let our countenances be looked upon before thee, and the countenance of the children that eat of the portion of the king's meat; and as thou seest, deal with thy servants.

So he consented to them in this matter, and proved them ten days.

And at the end of ten days their countenances appeared fairer and fatter in flesh than all the children which did eat the portion of the king's meat.

Thus Melzar took away the portion of their meat, and the wine that they should drink; and gave them pulse.

As for these four children, God gave them knowledge and skill in all learning and wisdom; and Daniel had under-

standing in all visions and dreams.

Now at the end of the days that the king had said he should bring them in, then the prince of the eunuchs brought them in before Nebuchadnezzar.

And the king communed with them; and among them all was found none like Daniel, Hananiah, Mishael, and Azariah; therefore stood they before the king.

And in all matters of wisdom and understanding, that the king inquired of them, he found them TEN TIMES BETTER than all the magicians and astrologers that were in all his realm.

And Daniel continued even unto the first year of king Cyrus.

Smith's Bible Dictionary (Philadelphia, 1948) defines *"pulse"* to usually mean peas, beans, and the seeds that grow in pods. In the Authorized Version it occurs only in Dan. 1:12, 16, as the translation of words the literal meaning of which is "seeds" of any kind. Probably the term denotes uncooked grain of any kind, as barley, wheat, millet, vetches, etc. (page 544).

Here then we have a unique situation in which Daniel was able to retain his identity by remaining "peculiar." He and his friends dared to be "different" because they loved the Lord more than they did man. They did not care to secure for themselves a popular image in Nebuchadnezzar's court. They were in Babylon, but desperately sought to not come part of her, as so many of their fellow Jews had done. They did not fall prey to "going along with the crowd" in eating the king's meat and drinking the king's wine. THEY BELIEVED IN CERTAIN HEALTH LAWS AND GOOD RULES OF NUTRITION and did not compromise these holy principles for the rich dainties and luscious fancies which the kitchens of Babylon could have yielded up to satisfy their hunger and soothe their appetites.

No! They maintained a position of peculiarity which was different than the rest of Israel in captivity at that time. It seems as if all the others forgot their God, and turned toward obeying the commandments of men instead. But, Daniel and his friends just could not compromise their love for God with the love for man. They could not substitute the one for the other. They felt they had to make a stand, declare their position, and then maintain it, even in the face of death.

The early Latter-day Saints were pretty much this way, too. They did not feel they should have to compromise good laws of health in order to satisfy the Gentiles in their mountain home with them. They did not believe in feeding their children the same kind of food which the Gentiles may have eaten; nor, did they feel to have such perishable commodities of refinement imported from the East either. They were "peculiar" because they believed in maintaining their own health standards as the Prophets had taught and encouraged them.

And one Gentile visitor, who happened through the territory in the early 1880's, was amazed at the results of the good nutritional habits practiced among the people in general:

> *Of the men in Orderville, I can say sincerely that a healthier, more stalwart community I have never seen, while among the women, I saw many refined faces, and remarked that robust health seemed the rule. Next morning the children were paraded, and such a brigade of infantry as it was! Their legs (I think, though they are known as 'limbs' in America) were positively columnar, and their chubby little owners were as difficult to keep quietly in line as so much quicksilver.* [10]

Another writer of about the same period remarked that "the faces of the Mormon children in the Deseret Sunday School Union are epitomes of good health and wise eating habits, unlike those of the pasty-white, emaciated figures back in the public schools of Boston." He then went on to describe their "ruddy-complexions," "lively step," "clear countenance," and "sparkling eyes." Surely, a noble tribute to such fine specimens of good health![11]

The Lord has given us, His people, a code of health by which to live. The Word of Wisdom is quite explicit about fresh fruits "in the season thereof," and green vegetables from the field. It also advises us how little we should eat meat—SPARINGLY! And the Doctrine and Covenants furnishes us with the key to correcting ill health—that if we have not faith, but believe, it is our privilege to be nourished back to health with herbs and mild food, as wisdom dictates.

Leading nutritional authorities throughout the country, not of our faith, have been proclaiming for years the harm in excessive use of refined foods, such as white flour, white sugar, processed cereals, artificial sweets, and soft-drinks. The author could fill ten more pages with enough evidence from these legitimate sources to prove his point, but shall avail himself of that for now, because it is not necessary to do.

However, the author does ask these questions: Have we, as God's People today, maintained a course in "peculiarity" which was similar to that of Daniel and his friends? Or, have we adopted some of the Gentile eating habits, to include in our diet, cola drinks, enriched bread products, excessive meat, refined-sugar, artificial sweets, etc.? Can we afford to ignore the laws of God in light of revealed wisdom? Should we conform ourselves to the same Gentile stupidity in nutrition and eating as plagues the rest of the world? Or, should we do as Daniel did, and maintain a course which is different than the one currently in vogue with Babylon? These are things to think about and seriously consider with an open mind and honest heart; for our life and health hang in the balance. And, if we are found wanting, who can venture to say what inevitable consequences we may have to suffer for our foolhardy actions?

Therefore, to be "peculiar" is not to rant and rave on health food, and be a belligerent fanatic about the same. But it is to maintain a quiet course of sensible living such as Apostle John A. Widstoe did while he was alive. When young, and in the old country, he would often go down to the fishing piers and help himself to a generous scoop of codliver oil from open barrels sitting around. And while in New York some years later, he was too poor to buy the expensive, enriched bread, so settled himself for the common, old "black bread," which was nothing more than the good wheat germ left over from the white flour used in the more costly loaves and dainty pastries; and this, according to his own daughter, too.

Brother Widstoe was the emblem of what good health and proper eating should be in any man. While others of his fellow apostles around him suffered from this problem or that trouble, he was going along as spry and nimble as a man in his busy position and advanced age could be.

John A. Widstoe was a dignified pillar of "peculiarity" and certainly kept alive in the Church during his time, that wonderful uniqueness of singularity, which has so marked Mormonism since its birth in 1830. The place of herbal medicine then, in the Church of Jesus Christ of Latter-day Saints, rests primarily with an individual, and becomes a personal sort of responsibility, rather a congregate sort of adaptation. If a person feels within himself to maintain that singular "peculiarity" which so marked the Prophet Joseph Smith, then it is his privilege and choice to so adopt those methods of the first great Seer and Revelator of this last Dispensation. On the other hand, if a man or woman wishes to go the way the rest of Judah went in Babylon, they should be allowed to do so while Daniel and his friends remain apart from the rest in their private habits and personal ways. But, it certainly is not for either one to condemn or judge the other in their chosen methods of action. For as Paul so beautifully put it: "Let not him that eateth despise him that eateth not; and let not him which eateth not judge him that eateth; for God hath received him."

NOTES

CHAPTER ONE

[1] Lucy Smith, Joseph Smith and his progenitors;Lamoni, Iowa, 1912; pp. 61-65.

[2]Calomel—so-called from its being white, though made from a dark mixture of mercury and corrosive sublimate. Mercurous chloride, HgCl, obtained as a fibrous crystalline mass or a white or yellowish-white powder by subliming a mixture of metallic mercury and corrosive sublimate, and in other ways. It is heavy, insoluble, and tasteless, and is much used in medicine as a mercurial purgative, and anthelmintic. (Webster's New International Dictionary of the English Language; 2nd Ed., unabridged; Massachusetts, 1946; p. 382).

[3] Ibid., pp. 97-100.

[4] Ibid., pp. 58-60.

CHAPTER TWO

[1] "Journal of Priddy Meeks," Utah Historical Quarterly 10:199.

Hereafter referred to as "Priddy Meeks" or "Quarterly," respectfully.

[2] Ibid., pp. 199-200.

[3] Ibid., pp. 149-150.

[4] Annals of Medical History, June 1925, in Utah Historical Society Library.

5 An agent which causes vomiting.

6 Eclectic—selecting; choosing what is thought best in doctrines, opinions, etc., from various sources or systems. Eclectism—(Medical). A system of medicine based on eclectic principles; specifically, U.S., one giving special attention to plant remedies. (Webster's, Ibid., p. 814).

7 Quarterly, op. cit., 10:44-48.

CHAPTER THREE

1 Alma 46:40.

2 "Medicine Among the Early Mormons;" an article by Claire Noall in the *California Folklore Quarterly* Vol. III, no. 2, April 1944; p. 158.

3 Doctrine & Covenants 42:43. Hereafter, cited as D&C.

4 D&C 89:10-11.

5 Webster's, op cit., p. 1166.

6 Ibid., p. 1014.

7 Priddy Meeks, op cit., pp. 213-214.

8 D&C 130:20-21.

9 Journals of Joseph Smith; October 5, 1835 entry; Church Historians Office, S.L.

10 Ibid., Sat. October 10, 1835.

11 D&C 42:44.

12 "Medicine and the Mormons;" an article by Robert T. Divett, in the *Bulletin of the Medical Library Association*; Vol. 31, No. 1, January 1936; p. 3. Hereafter, cited as "Direct" in this work.

13 Dirk J. Struik, *Yankee Science in the Making*; Boston, 1948; pp. 176-178.

14 Noall, op cit., pp. 159-160.

15 Franklin L. West, Life of Franklin D. Richards; 1924; p. 15.

16 2 Nephi 4:34.

17 Ibid.

18 John 14:15.

CHAPTER FOUR

1*The Songs of Zion*; Chicago, 1908; p. 9.

2 *Documentary History of the Church*; Salt Lake City, 1908; Volume 4; pp. 70-71. Hereafter cited in this work as DHC.

3 Genesis 1:31.

4 Ibid., 3:24.

5 Matthew 13:17.

6 Mark 4:21-26.

7 Romans 14:1-3.

8 DHC 4:414 (September 5, 1841).

9 Journals of Joseph Smith, op. cit., December 29, 1842 entry.

10 Henry Caswall, *The City of the Mormons or Three Days at Nauvoo in 1842*; London, 1842.

11 Journals of Joseph Smith, op cit.

12 Divett, op cit., pp. 2-3.

[13] Caswall, op cit., p. 16.

[14] Minutes of the Female Relief Society of Nauvoo, March 17, 1842 - March 16, 1844. L.D.S. Church Historian's Office, Salt Lake City, Utah.

[15] "Pioneer Midwives" by Kate Carter; DUP Lesson for April, 1963; op. 429-430.

[16] Noall, op cit., p. 161.

[17] Utah Historical Quarterly, op cit., pp. 34-35.

[18] From an oral interview conducted by the author personally, in the Summer of 1972, with Mrs., Orem, Utah; whose request it was to remain anonymous when so quoted later on. Name and material in possession of the author, Manti, Utah.

[18a] "Superstitions, Customs, and Prescriptions of Mormon Midwives;" an article by Claire Noall; *California Historical Quarterly*, 3:103-104; 108; April, 1944.

[19] West, op cit., p. 15.

[20] Quarterly, op cit., pp. 32-33.

[21] Noall, op cit., p. 157; 164.

[22] Quarterly, op cit., p. 42.

[23] 2 Corinthians 3:6

[24] The Far West Record; entry for August 31, 1834. L.D.S. Church Historian's Office, Salt Lake City.

[25] Priddy Meeks, op cit., pp. 1880-81.

[26] Jared Carter Journals (Jan. 1831-Jan. 26, 1833). Church Historian's Office, Salt Lake City.

[27] Joseph Fielding Smith, *Teachings of the Prophet Joseph Smith*; Salt Lake City, 1940; p. 321.

[28] The Songs of Zion, op cit., p. 9.

CHAPTER FiVE

[1] Archival material in possession of the author, Manti, Utah.

[2] Jethro Kloss, Back to Eden; Tennessee, 1939; p. 253.

[3] lbid., pp. 253-254.

[4] Priddy Meeks, op cit., pp. 175-176.

[5] lbid., p. 215.

[6] Ibid., p. 185.

[7] lbid., p. 199.

[8] Ibid., pp. 197-198.

[9] Ibid., pp. 174-175.

[10] Quarterly, op cit., p. 38.

[11] Ibid., pp. 38-39.

[12] Nels Anderson, Deseret Saints—The Mormon Frontier in Utah; Chicago, 1942; pp. 356-7.

[13] Priddy Meeks, op cit., p. 213.

[14] Ibid., p. 185.

CHAPTER SIX

[1] An apocryphal work, in no way connected with the canonized or accepted versions of the Bible now in use in Christendom.

[2] Douglas Guthrie, A History of Medicine; 1946; pp. 29-30.

[3] Lucy Mack Smith, op cit., pp. 948-49.

[4] Isaiah 55:8-9.

[5] N.B. Lundwall, Faith Like the Ancients; Salt Lake City, 1950;

pp. 60-64.

6 The "Hall System" of cure advocated the constant use of colon flushing (or the administration of frequent enemas) as a means of proper bowel elimination, to prevent constipation; and, otherwise avoid any serious attack of appendicitis which may develop.

7 Benjamin F. Johnson, My Life 'a Review;' Independence, Missouri, 1947; p. 61.

8 A History of George Spilsbury, by himself; p. 3. Special Collections, Harold B. Lee Library, Brigham Young University, Provo, Utah.

9 Hubert Howe Bancroft, History of Utah; Salt Lake CIty, 1964; p. 233.

10 Memoirs of John R. Young, by himself; Salt Lake City, 1920; p. 64.

11 B. F. Johnson, op. cit., pp. 109-111.

12 Kloss, op. cit., p. 171.

13 The Diary of Isaiah Moses Coombs (Beaver, Utah). A typescript copy in the possession of the author.

14 Priddy Meeks, op. cit., pp. 210-211.

15 "Medicine In The Bible;" A Sketch of Medicine and Pharmacy by Samuel Evans Massengill, Mdl.; Bristol, Tennessee, 1943; p. 253.

16 Exodus 30:35.

17 Frederick M. Rossiter, B.S., M.D., *The Practical Guide to Health*; California, 1913; p. 221.

18 Ibid., title-page; under the author's respective name, are his accreditations listed.

19 Dr. Frank McCoy, The Past Way To Health; Los Angeles, 1926; pp. 120-122.

20 George C. Lantert, Precious Memories; (Sixteenth Book of the Faith-Promoting Series); Salt Lake City, 1974; pp. 12-13.

[21] Juvenile Instructor 35:764.

[22] Songs of Zion, op. cit., hymn no. 155.

CHAPTER SEVEN

[1] Journal History; entry for August 19, 1846. Church Library, Salt Lake City.

[2] Ibid.

[3] Archival material in author's possession.

[4] Daniel Tyler, *A Concise History of the Mormon Battalion in the Mexican War* (1846—184?); 1881; pp. 127-128.

[5] lbid., p. 147.

[6] lbid p. 183.

[7] J. V. Long, *Report of The First General Festival of The Renowned Mormon Battalion*; St. Louis, 1855; pp. 28; 33. (Rare pamphlet in Church Library, Salt Lake City.)

[8] Divett, op. cit., p. 5.

[9] Deseret News, January 20, 1858.

[10] Quarterly, op. cit., pp. 42-43.

[11] Ibid., p. 42.

[12] Journals of Wilford Woodruff (August-September, 1842 entry); Church Historian's Office, Salt Lake City, Utah.

[13] Two references for this: (a) Documentary History of the Church 5:60-61. Friday, July 1,5 1842.—It was reported early in the morning that Elder Orson Pratt was missing. I caused the Temple hands and the principal men of the city to make search for him .... Elder Pratt returned in the evening. (b) Thomas Edgar Lyon, *Orson Pratt—Early Mormon Leader*; University of Chicago Dissertation, M.A. ; June, 1932; p. 29. Ebenezer Robinson, an associate editor of the Times and Seasons

said Pratt was found 5 miles below Nauvoo, in a state of frenzy sitting on the bank of the Mississippi River.

[14] Woodruff, op. cit., entry for Sept. 24, 1865, 1860-65 Bk.

[15] Quarterly, op. cit., p. 21.

[16] Kate Carter, "Pioneer Midwives," DUP Lesson for April, 1963; p. 483.

[17] Ibid., May, 1963; p. 504.

[18] Priddy Meeks, op. cit., pp. 178-179.

[19] Quarterly, op cit., p. 38.

[20] An early Jaredite name, signifying "honeybee," appropriated to Utah by the Mormons before it achieved statehood.

[21] Quarterly, op. cit., p. 39.

[22] Priddy Meeks, its first President, had removed himself to Parowan, Utah, and thus was unable to continue officiating in that capacity, and had to relinquish his office and title to another.

[23] Quarterly, op. cit., p. 13.

[24] Claire Noall, *Intimate Disciple*; University of Utah Press, 1957; pp. 574; 620.

[25] Ibid., p. 575.

[26] Kate B. Carter, "Pioneer Women Doctors," DUP Lesson for March, 1963; p. 363.

[27] Quarterly, op. cit., p. 43.

[28] Divett, op. cit., p. 8.

[29] Rose, Blanche E., "Early Utah Medical Practice;" *Utah Historical Quarterly* 10:22-25.

[30] Richards, Ralph 1., *Of Medicine, Hospitals, and Doctors*; Salt Lake City, 1953; p. 23.

[31] Noall, Claire Wilcox, "Utah's Pioneer Women Doctors;"

Improvement Era, 42:16-17 ff.

32 Rose, Blanche, *The History of Medicine in Utah*; an unpublished master's thesis in the University of Utah Medical Library; Salt Lake City, 1939; pp. 75-78.

33 Noall, Era, op. cit., pp. 144-145 ff.

34 An oral Interview with Elvira Dastrup, Richfield, Utah; granddaughter of Patriarch Elias H. Blackburn. Interview conducted by the author's father and brother, Jacob and Joseph Heinerman, August 8, 1973, in the home of Sister Dastrup. A full account of this hour-long interview is in the possession of the author, Manti, Utah.

35 Journal of Discourses 14:230. Hereafter referred to as JD.

36 This prophecy has been literally fulfilled in modern times; for there is not a woman in the Church today, hardly, who will not submit herself into the hands of a doctor and be placed under his care during the final stages of pregnancy, prior to delivery. However, it is noteworthy to relate that in recent years, certain prominent people in America have begun to adapt themselves more to a course of health foods, herbal medicine, and midwifery than has ever been found to be the custom before. Actors such as Dennis Weaver and Robert Curnings are staunch advocates of health foods and some herbal teas. Actresses such as Susan Oliver and Anita Bryant believe in the same things, plus natural childbirth at home. Among many of the middle-class, it has become the thing in vogue to have children right at home, with the assistance of a qualified mid-wife in attendance. Such books as *Foxfire One* and *Foxfire Two*, give useful information on mid-wifery and even provide for chapters on herbal remedies of the Ozark Mountain folk in Kentucky. Popular works, like "The Whole Earth Catalogue" make specific mention of both mid-wifery and herbal medicine, and give places where such might be purchased or courses obtained in the same. It seems to be a national fad of late, for these sort of things; kind of a "return to nature" amidst the scientific technology of our civilization.

37 JD 15:225-226.

38 Richards, op. cit., p. 15.

39 An oath, embodying an admirable code of medical ethics, generally taken by young men about to begin medical practice, said to have been imposed by Hippocrates on his disciples.

40 Quarterly, op. cit., p. 48.

41 Ibid.

CHAPTER EIGHT

1 *The Deseret News*, October 24, 1855. Also quoted in: J. Cecil Altar, *Utah the Storied Domain*; Vol. 1, p. 210.

2 JD 23:189-195.

3 Juvenile Instructor 28:669, an editorial.

4 Deseret Weekly News 49:449-450, 451. Sermon given in the Millcreek Ward, Salt Lake.

5 Young Woman's Journal 2:278-280.

6 Ibid., 2:32.

7 Relief Society Bulletin, Vol. 1, no. 1, pp. 5-6.

8 Jeremiah Stokes, *Modern Miracles*; pp. 149-150.

9 Minnie I. Hodapp, *Book of Remembrance* (The Christian Olsen Family, 1821-1950); Provo, Utah, December, 1950; privately printed; pp. 79-80.

10 Kate B. Carter, "Pioneer Women Doctors;" DUP Lesson for March, 1963; p. 396.

11 Ibid., p. 409.

12 Kate B. Carter, "Pioneer Midwives;" DUP Lesson for May, 1963; pp. 543-544.

13 Ibid., p. 551.

14 Richards, op. cit., pp. 16-17;80.

15 Autobiography of Violet Ure; Church Historian's Office, Salt Lake City, Utah.

16 Gene A. Sessions, Mormon Democrat—*The Religious and Political Memoirs of James Henry Moyle*; typescript prepared under the direction of the Historical Department of The Church of Jesus Christ of Latter-day Saints; 1975; pp. 11-12. Available in the Church library downstairs, Salt Lake City, Utah.

CHAPTER NINE

1 Dr. James D. Allen and Dr. Richard O. Cowan, *Mormonism In The Twentieth Century*; Brigham Young University Press, Provo, Utah; 1969; p. 66.

2 *The New York Spectator*; Tuesday, September 21, 1831; as quoted from a Missouri newspaper by them. An original copy is in the possession of the author.

3 Hector Lee, *The Three Nephites;* The University of New Mexico Press, Albuquerque; 1949; p. 120.

4 Nels Anderson, *Desert Saints*; Chicago, 1942; pp. 443, 445.

5 "History of Martha Mariah Myers Hancock;" pp. 18-19; 22-23. A typescript copy of the original, in the possession of the author's father, Manti, Utah.

6 Taken from an oral interview, with his daughter, Ann Wallis, of Salt Lake City, at the old University of Utah Library. Interview conducted by the author's father, Jacob Heinerman, in 1952, who was a personal acquaintance of Sister Wallis, and knew her very well. Typescript copy in possession of the author's father, Manti, Utah.

7 Mark 16:16-19.

8 Archival material in the possession of the author.

9 Diary of Emily Dow Partridge Young; pp. 55-56. Special Collections, Harold B. Lee Library, Brigham Young University, Provo, Utah.

10 Phil Robinson, *Sinners and Saints*; Boston, 1883; pp. 233-234.

11 Archival material in possession of the author.

APPENDIX A

HERB TABLE

(A List of Herbs Mentioned in This Work; Their Various Names,
Descriptions, and Medicinal Properties)

The following plants and their characteristics are taken from the book
Back to Eden by Jethro Kloss, Herbalist (Tennessee, 1967).

BAYBERRY
(Bark, Leaves, and Flowers)

Botanical name: Myrica Cerifera. Common names: Bayberry
Bush, American Bayberries, American vegetable tallow tree, Bayberry
wax tree, Myrtle, wax myrtle, candleberry, candleberry myrtle, tallow
shrub, American vegetable wax, vegetable tallow. Medicinal properties:
Astringent, tonic, stimulant. Leaves: Aromatic, stimulant.

One of the most valuable and useful herbs. The tea is a most
excellent gargle for sore throat. It will thoroughly cleanse the throat of all
putrid matter. Steep a teaspoonful in a pint of boiling water for thirty
minutes, gargle the throat thoroughly until it is clean, then drink a pint
lukewarm to thoroughly cleanse the stomach. If it does not come back
easily, tickle the back of the throat. This restores the mucous secretions to
normal activity. For chills, make as above, adding a pinch of Cayenne, and
take a half cup warm every hour. This is very effective.

Bayberry is excellent to take as an emetic after narcotic poisoning
of any kind, and it is good to follow with a lobelia emetic.

Bayberry is valuable taken in the usual manner for all kinds of
hemorrhages, whether from the stomach, lungs, uterus, or bowels.
Bayberry is reliable to check profuse menstruation, and when combined

with Capsicum is an unfailing remedy for this. Very good in leucorrhea. Has an excellent general effect on the female organs, also has an excellent influence on the uterus in pregnancy, and makes a good douche. Excellent results will be obtained from its use in goitre. In diarrhea and dysentery, use an injection of the tea as an enema.

In case of gangrene sores, boils, carbuncles, use as a wash and poultice, or apply the powdered bayberry to the infection. The tea is an excellent wash for spongy and bleeding gums.

Bayberry is an excellent treatment in adenoids by snuffing the powder or tea up the nose, or using a straw through which to blow the powdered bayberry. This is also good for catarrh.

The tea taken internally is useful in jaundice, scrofula, canker in the throat and mouth. The tea taken warm promotes perspiration, and improves the whole circulation, and tones up the tissues. Taken in combination with yarrow, catnip, sage or peppermint, is unexcelled for colds.

An excellent formula used by the famous Dominion Herbal College made with bayberry for colds, fevers, flu, colic, cramps, and pains in the stomach is as follows:

Bayberry	4 oz.
Ginger	2 oz.
White Pine	1 oz.
Cloves	1 dram
Capsicum	1 dram

This is prepared by mixing the herbs (in powdered form) and passing through a fine sieve several times. Use one teaspoonful more or less as the case may require, in a cup of hot water. Allow the herbs to stand so they will settle and drink off the clear liquid, leaving the settlings. Anyone knowing the benefit of this wonderful composition would not be without it.

BALMONY

Botanical name: Chelone glabra. Common names: Snake head, turtlebloom, turtle head, salt rheurn weed, fishmouth shell flower, bitter herb. Medicinal properties: Tonic, antibilious stimulant, detergent, authelmintic.

Specific tonic for enfeebled stomach and indigestion, general debility and biliousness, juandice, constipation dyspepsia, and torpid liver. Almost a certain remedy for worms. Increase the gastric and salivary secretions and stimulates the appetite. Good for sores and eczema.

BITTERROOT
(Root)

Botanical name: Apocynum androsaemifolium. Common names: Dogsbane, milkweed, honey bloom, milk ipecac, flytrap, wandering mildweed, catchfly, bitter dogsbanes, western wallflower. Medical properties: Emetic, diuretic, sudonific, cathartic, stimulant, expectorant.

This is a very good remedy for intermittent fever, typhoid fever, and other fevers. Has an excellent effect on the liver, kidneys, and bowels. Increases the secretion of bile. Excellent for poor digestion. Bitterroot has been known to cure dropsy when everything else has failed. Expels worms. Is very useful in syphilis, and to rid the system of other impurities. Especially valuable in gallstones. Good in rheumatism, neuralgia, diseases of the joints and mucous membranes. Wonderful for diabetes.

BURDOCK
(Root, Leaves, and Seeds)

Botanical name: Arctium lappa. Common names: Grass burdock, clotbur, bandana, burr seed, hardock, harebur, hurrburr, turkey burr seed. Medicinal properties: Root: Diuretic, depilatory, alterative. Leaves: Maturing. Seed: Alternative, diuretic.

The root is one of the best blood purifiers for syphilitic and other diseases of the blood. It cleanses and eliminates impurities from the blood very rapidly. Burdock tea taken freely will clear all kinds of skin diseases, boils, and carbuncles. Increases flow of urine. Excellent for gout, rheumatism, scrofula, canker sores, syphilis, sciatica, gonorrhea, leprosy. Wring a hot fomentation out of the tea for swellings. It is good to make a salve and apply externally for skin eruptions, burns, wounds, swellings, and hemorrhoids. Excellent to reduce flesh.

CATNIP

Botanical name: Nepeta cataria. Common names: Catmint, catrup, cat's-wort, field balm, catnip. Medicinal properties: Anodyne, antispasmodic, carmintative, aromatic, diaphoretic, nervine.

Catnip is one of the oldest household remedies. It is wonderful for very small children and infants. Use the tea as an injection for children in convulsions. Very useful in pain of any kind, spasms, wind colic, excellent to allay gas, acids in stomach and bowels, prevent griping. A tablespoonful steeped in a pint of water used as an enema is soothing and quieting, and very effective in insanity, fevers, expelling worms in children; also fits. A high enema of catnip will relieve hysterical headaches. It is good to restore menstrual secretions. Catnip, sweet balm, marshmellow and sweet weed make an excellent baby remedy. If mothers would have this on hand and use it properly, it would save them many sleepless nights and doctor's bills, and also save the baby much suffering. It is a harmless remedy and should take the place of the various soothing syrups on the market, many of which are very harmful. This wonderful remedy should be in every home. A little honey or malt honey may be added to make it palatable. Steep, never boil, catnip. Take internally freely. An enema of catnip will cause urination when it has stopped.

CAYENNE PEPPER
(Fruit)

Botanical name: Capsicum annuum. Common names: Cayenne pepper, red pepper, capsicum, Spanish pepper, bird pepper, pod pepper, chillies, African pepper, chili pepper, African red pepper, cockspur pepper, American red pepper, garden pepper. Medicinal properties: Pungent, stimulant, tonic, sialagogue, alterative,

Red pepper is one of the most wonderful herb medicines we have. We do wonderful things with it that we are not able to do with any other known herb. It should never be classed with black pepper, vinegar, or mustard. These are irritating, while red pepper is very soothing. While red pepper smarts a little, it can be put in an open wound, either in a fresh wound, or an old ulcer, and it is very healing instead of irritating; but black pepper, mustard, and vinegar are irritating to an open wound and do not heal. Red pepper is one of the most stimulating herbs known to man with no harm or reaction.

It is effective as a poultice for rheumatism, inflamation, pleurisy, and helpful also if taken internally for these. For sores and wounds it makes a good poultice. It is a stimulant when taken internally as well as being antispasmodic. Good for kidneys, spleen, and pancreas. Wonderful for lockjaw. Will heal a sore, ulcerated stomach; while black pepper, mustard, or vinegar will irritate it. Red pepper is a specific and very effective remedy in yellow fever, as well as other fevers and may be taken in capsules followed by a glass of water.

It is one part of a most wonderful liniment, which may be made as follows:

2 oz. gum myrrh
1 oz. golden seal
1/2 oz. African red pepper

Put this into a quart of rubbing alcohol, or take a pint of raspberry vinegar and a pint of water. Add the alcohol or vinegar to the power. Let it stand for a week or ten days, shaking every day. This can be used wherever liniment is useful or needed. It is very healing to wounds, bruises, sprains, scalds, burns, and sunburns, and should be applied freely. Wonderful results are obtained in pyorrhea by rinsing the mouth with the liniment or applying the liniment on both sides of the gums with a little cotton or gauze.

CINNAMON AND CLOVES

Spices which may be purchased in any local food market. Available in ground powder, whole, or stick.

Cinnamon is delicious used in baked or fried apples, apple sauce, apple pies and dumplings. Use in waffles, muffins, coffee cakes, pancakes, cookies, and French toast. Mix with sugar for cinnamon toast or sprinkle over cupcakes before baking. Add to grilled bananas and stewed fruit, such as prunes, pears and peaches. Excellent in custards and rice pudding.

The stick cinnamon is a delightful addition to hot apple cider.

When ready to serve, add a piece and stir with a spoon. Leave the stick in and it will give a unique and wonderful flavor to the beverage.

Powdered cloves can be used in preparing fruit cake, plum pudding, apple pie, steamed puddings, bread puddings, pumpkin pie, cookies, cranberries, glazes for ham and other meats, spice cake, gingerbread, mincemeat, frostings, spiced nuts, coffee cake, sweet rolls, streusel toppings, broiled bananas and grapefruit, chili sauce, tomato relish, carrots, squash, sweet potatoes and onions.

Whole cloves may be inserted into a ham, prior to baking. Make light slashes on both sides of the ham about an inch or so apart, in kind of a criss-cross effect, and put a small piece of clove into each tiny square. It gives the ham a delicious flavor.

Powdered cinnamon may be sprinkled on rolled oats before cooking, to make it an additional breakfast treat for youngsters.

Measure out the proper amount of rolled oats you wish to use; put in the appropriate water (use cold); add a dab of butter or margarine; and then shake on a little cinnamon. Stir together; set on stove; cover; and cook over medium heat. Stir occasionally to prevent from sticking. Serve hot with milk.

GOLDEN SEAL
(Root)

Botanical name: Hydrastis canadensis. Common names: Yellow paint root, orange root, yellow puccoon, ground raspberry, eye root, yellow Indian paint, Indian plant, tumenic root, Ohio curcuma, eye balm, yellow eye, jaundice root. Medicinal properties: Laxative, tonic, alterative, detergent, opthalmicum, antiperiodic, aperient, diuretic, antiseptic, deobstruent.

This is one of the most wonderful remedies in the entire herb kingdom. When it is considered all that can be accomplished by its use, and what it actually will do, it does seem like a cure-all.

It is one of the best substitutes for quinine, is a most excellent remedy for colds, la grippe, and all kinds of stomach and liver troubles. It exerts a special influence on all the mucous membranes and tissues with which it comes in contact. For open sores, inflammations, eczema, ringworm, erysipelas, or any skin disease, golden seal excels. Golden seal tea is made by steeping one teaspoonful in a pint of boiling water for twenty minutes and used as a wash, then after the place is thoroughly clean (it is well to use peroxide of hydrogen for cleansing). Sprinkle some of the powdered root and cover. Taken in small but frequent doses, it will allay nausea during pregnancy. Steep a teaspoonful in a pint of boiling water for twenty minutes, stir well, let settle, and pour off the liquid. Take six tablespoonfuls a day. It equalizes the circulation and combined with scullcap and red pepper (cayenne) will greatly relieve and strengthen the heart. It has no superior when combined with myrrh, one part golden seal to one-fourth myrrh for ulcerated stomach, duodenum, dyspepsia, and is especially good for enlarged tonsils and sores in the mouth. Smoker's sores, caused by holding a pipe in the mouth, will heal after just a few applications of the powder to the sore. I have used it in a number of cases that were called "skin cancers" with excellent results.

It is an excellent remedy for diphtheria, tonsillitis, and other serious throat troubles, and has a good effect combined with a little myrrh and cayenne. Excellent for chronic catarrh of the intestines and all catarrhal conditions. Will improve appetite and aid digestion. Combined with scullcap and hops, it is a very fine tonic for spinal nerves; is very good in spinal meningitis. Very useful in all skin eruptions, scarlet fever, and smallpox.

To cure pyorrhea or sore gums, put a little of the tea in a cup, dip the toothbrush in it, and thoroughly brush the teeth and gums. The results will be most satisfactory. In any nose trouble, pour some tea in the hollow of the hand and snuff up the nose. Very useful in typhoid fever, gonorrhead, leucorrhea and syphilis. For bladder troubles, it should be injected into the bladder immediately after the bladder has been emptied, and retained as long as possible, repeating two or three times a day. I do not recomend that individuals do this for themselves unless experienced. Have a physician or nurse inject it for you with a rubber catheter.

Golden seal combined with alum root, taken internally, is an excellent remedy for bowel and bladder troubles. Use two parts of golden seal and one part wild alum. This is a laxative. Good for piles, hemorrhoids, and prostate gland. When combined with equal parts of red clover blossoms, yellow dock, and dandelion it has a wonderful effect on the gall bladder, liver, pancreas, spleen, and kidneys. Combined with peach leaves, queen of the meadow, cleavers and corn silk, it is a reliable remedy for Bright's disease and diabetes. Golden seal is excellent for the eyes. The following is the way the writer uses it for his eyes: Steep a small teaspoonful of golden seal and one of boric acid in a pint of boiling water, stir thoroughly, let cool, and pour liquid off. Put a teaspoonful of this liquid in a half cup of water. Bathe the eyes with this, using an eye cup, or drop it in with an eye dropper. If the eyelids are granulated or there is film over the eyes, add one teaspoonful burnt alum powder. If you use it a little too strong, there is no harm done; it will only smart a little. Golden seal may be taken in different ways, and may be used alone in all cases given above where it is suggested to combine with others. Take one-fourth teaspoonful of golden seal dissolved in a glass of hot water immediately upon arising, a glass one hour before noon and evening meal. Of you may steep a teaspoonful in a pint of boiling water, stir thoroughly, let cool, pour liquid off and take a tablespoon four to six times a day. Children should take less of all doses according to age.

There are many remedies much advertised as containing golden seal, but the fact is, there is so little golden seal in the preparations, that it does very little good, as it is very expensive.

Chronic catarrh of the intestines, even to the extent of ulceration, is greatly benefited by golden seal. Golden seal produces healing in ulceration of the mucous lining of the rectum, effectual in hemorrhage of the rectum. It is a remedy for chronic and intermittent malarial poisoning or enlarged spleen of malarial origin. From the above it will be seen how applicable golden seal is in all catarrhal conditions, whether of the throat, nasal passages, bronchial tubes, intestines, stomach, bladder, or wherever there is a lining of mucous membrane. It kills poisons.

HOREHOUND
(Plant)

Botanical name: Marrubium volgare. Common names: Horehound, white horehound. Medicinal properties: Pectoral, aromatic, diaphoretic, tonic, expectorant, diuretic, hepatic stimulant.

Horehound will produce profuse perspiration when taken hot. Taken in large doses, it is a laxative. When taken cold, is good for dyspepsia, jaundice, asthema, hysteria, and will expel worms. Very useful in chronic sore throat, coughs, consumption, and all pulmonary infections. If the menses stop abnormally, it will bring them back. Horehound is one of the old-fashioned remedies and should be in every home ready for immediate use. Horehound syrup is excellent for asthma and difficult breathing. For children in coughs or croup, steep a heaping tablespoonful in a pint of boiling water for twenty minutes, strain, add honey, and let them take freely.

INDIGO ROOT

Not too common as an herb today. There are several types of indigo plants from which a blue dye is obtained by extraction. Nothing is given in Back To Eden about it. Apparently, the pioneers were more familiar with it than modern herbalists are.

MAGNOLIA
(Bark)

Botanical name: Magnolia glauca. Common names: Swamp laurel, red laurel, sweet magnolia, red bay, white bay beaver tree, Indian bark, sweet bay, swamp sassafras, holly bay. Medical properties: Astringent, stimulant, febrifuge, tonic aromatic, anti-periodic.

This is an excellent tonic, very valuable in intermittent fever, dyspepsia, dysentery, and erysipelas. Use as a douche for leucorrhea. A wash made by simmering a tablespoonful of magnolia bark in a pint of water for ten minutes is fine for salt rheum and other skin diseases. Magnolia is excellent to use in place of quinine, and will do the work when quinine falls. Effective to cure the tobacco habit. This herb can be taken a long time without any bad effects.

PENNYROYAL
(Whole Plant)

Botanical name: Hedeoina Pulegioides. Common names: Tickweed, squaw mint, stinking balm, thickweed, American pennyroyal. Medicinal properties: Sudoriflc carminative, eninenagogue, stimulant, diaphoretic, aromatic, sedative.

Is excellent in burning fevers. Will promote perspiration. Take hot. Excellent remedy for toothache, gout, leprosy, colds, consumption, phlegm in chest and lungs, jaundice, dropsy, cramps, convulsions, headache, ulcers, sores in mouth, insect and snake bites, itch, intestinal pains, colic, and griping. If trouble with suppressed or scanty menstruation, take one or two cupfuls hot at bedtime along with a hot foot bath, several days before expected. It will relieve nausea, but should not be taken by a pregnant woman. Good as a poultice, and wash for bruises, black-eye. Good for nervousness and hysteria, useful for skin diseases.

PEPPERMINT

Botanical name: Mentha piperita. Medicinal properties: Aromatic, stimulant, stomachic, carminative. Oil: Stimulant, rubfacient.

This is one of the oldest household remedies and should be in every garden, as it grows very prolifically. Excellent remedy for chills, colic, fevers, dizziness or, gas in stomach, nausea, vomiting, diarrhea, dysentery, cholera, heart trouble, palpitation of the heart, influenza, la grippe and hysteria. Applied externally is good for rheumatism, neuralgia and headache. Peppermint enemas are excellent for cholera and colon troubles. It is helpful in cases of insanity, and especially useful for convulsions and spasms in infants.

Peppermint is a general stimulant. A strong cup of peppermint tea will act more powerfully on the system than any liquor stimulant, quickly diffusing itself through the system and bringing back to the body its natural warmth in itself through the system and bringing back to the body its natural warmth in case of sudden fainting or dizzy spells, with extreme coldness and pale countenance.

Will bring back to the body its natural warmth and glow without the usual tendency to relapse. Good for gripping pain caused by eating unripe fruit or irritating foods.

Do not drink coffee and tea, which are so harmful. Coffee weakens the heart muscles—peppermint tea is delicious and strengthens your heart muscles. Coffee hinders digestion, weakens the heart, is one cause of constipation, poisons the body. Peppermint tea cleanses and strengthens the entire body. Give it a fair trial and see how much better you feel when you leave off coffee and tea and drink peppermint tea.

In place of aspirin for the headache, or any other harmful headache drug, take a cup of as-strong-as-you-like-it peppermint tea, lie down for a little while, and see what a good effect it will have. If need be, drink two or three cups, or enough so it gets into the system so it can help you, and it will not disappoint you. Strengthens the nerves instead of weakening them as aspirin, and other drugs do.

If the tea is not at hand, take some of the leaves and chew them up fine until you can swallow them easily. This will start the food to digesting and assist the entire system to do its work more normally.

PIG WEED

Nothing given on it.

PLEURISY ROOT
(Root)

Botanical name: Asclepias tuberosa. Common names: Butterfly weed, wind root, Canada root, silkweed, orange swallow wort, tuber root, white root, flux root, asclepias. Medicinal properties: Expectorant, carminative, tonic, diuretic, diaphoretic, relaxant, antispasmodic.

As the name suggests, it is very valuable in pleurisy. Excellent to break up colds, for la grippe, and all bronchial and pulmonary complaints. Very useful in scarlet fever, rheumatic fevers, lung fever, bilious fever, typhus, and all burning fevers, also measles. Good for suppressed menstruation and acute dysentery.

Treatment of pleurisy: Clean the stomach out first with an emetic. Steep a teaspoonful of powdered pleurisy root in a cup of boiling water for forty-five minutes, strain, and take two tablespoonfuls every two hours—oftener, if necessary. Apply to the affected part a cold compress, covering well with a flannel. Give a high enema of pleurisy root, using a tablespoonful to a quart of boiling water. Let steep and use about 112° F.

It is a tonic for the kidneys. Good for asthma.

POPLAR
(Bark and Leaves)

Botanical name: Populus tremuloides. Common names: Aspen, American aspen, quaking aspen, quaking asp, quiver leaf, trembling tree, treetling poplar, white poplar, aspen poplar, abele tree. Medicinal properties: Stomachi, febrifuge, tonic, antiperiodic.

Poplar is better than quinine for all purposes for which quinine is used. Very useful for diseases of urinary organs, especially if weak. Excellent to aid digestion and to tone up run-down condition, either in disease or old age. Very good in all cases of diarrhea. Excellent for acute rheumatism. Good in all fevers, such as intermittent fever, influenza, etc. Good for neuralgia, la grippe, jaundice, liver and kidney trouble, diabetes, hay fever, cholera infantum. Will expel worms. Is splendid used externally as a wash for cancer, bad ulcers, gangrenous wounds, eczema, strong perspiration, burns and sores caused by gonorrhea and syphilis. It is more effective than quinine in fever and la grippe.

RED RASPBERRY
(Leaves and Fruit)

Botanical name: Rubus stringosus. Common names: Wild red raspberry, raspberry. Medicinal properties: Leaves: Anti-emetic, astringent, purgative, stomachic, parturient, tonic, stimulant, alterative. Fruit: Laxative, exculent, anti-acid, parturient.

Will remove cankers from mucous membrane. Excellent for dysentery and diarrhea, especially in infants. It decreases the menstrual flow without abruptly stopping it. Is very soothing and does not excite. Good to combine in such cases with prickly ash, blue cohosh, wild yam, and cinnamon. Will allay nausea. When the bowels are greatly relaxed, use in place of coffee and tea.

RHUBARB
(Root)

Botanical name: Rheum palmatium. Common names: Turkey rhubarb, China rhubarb. Medicinal properties: Vulnerary, tonic, stomachic, purgative, astringent, aperient.

Rhubarb is an old-time remedy, very useful for diarrhea and dysentery in adults and children. An excellent laxative for infants, as it is very mild and tonic. Excellent to increase the muscular action of the bowels. Excellent for use in stomach troubles. Will relieve headache. It stimulates the gall-ducts, thereby causing the ejection of bilious materials. Excellent for scrofulous children with distended abdomens. Good for the liver. Cleans and tones the bowels.

SAGE
(Leaves)

Botanical name: Saliva officinalis. Common name: Garden sage. Medicinal properties: Sudorific, astringent, expectorant, tonic, aromatic, antispasmodic, nervine, vermifuge.

Sage is a well-known seasoning for roasts, soups, etc. The tea is an excellent gargle for ulcerated throat or mouth. It can be mixed with a little lemon and honey. An excellent article for excessive sexual desire and sexual debility. One of the best remedies for stomach troubles, dyspepsia, gas in the stomach, and bowels. For quinsy, take the tea externally and also gargle the throat. Will expel worms in adults and children. Will stop bleeding of wounds, very cleansing to old ulcers and sores. Good for spermatorrhea. Also in liver and kidney troubles. Wounds of any kind will heal more rapidly when washed with sage tea. It is very soothing in nervous troubles and delirious fevers. A most effective hair tonic. Will make hair grow when the roots are not destroyed, and remove dandruff. As a substitute for quinine, it is better than this drug.

For fever, la grippe, or pneumonia, first take a high enema; next take a big dose of body cleanser and laxative. Then go to bed and take three, four, or five cups of hot sage tea in short intervale—say a half hour apart. This will cause free perspiration, will make the whole body active, and will throw off the cold. It will relieve the pains in the head. It produces strong circulation. A strong tea is excellent to gargle for sore throat. This tea, drunk cold during the day, will prevent night sweats.

The American people would do well if they would use sage instead of tea and coffee. The Chinese make fun of the American people because they buy the expensive tea for their drink and pay a big price for it, while the Chinese buy sage from America for a small price and drink that for their tea, which is a most wonderful remedy. The Chinese know that the sage tea will keep them well, while the tea that we buy from the Chinese makes the American people sick, is a cause of great nervousness and one of the causes of insanity. Sage tea is very soothing and quieting to the nerves, while the tea that we buy from China is a great cause of nervousness, headache, and delirium. In case of weaning a child, or when it is desired that the milk should cease in the breasts, in case of sickness or other reasons, the sage tea, drunk cold, will cause the flow of milk in the breasts to cease.

This tea should not be boiled, but just steeped. It should be kept covered while steeping. The ordinary dose is a heaping teaspoonful to a cup of hot water. Let it steep twenty or thirty minutes. Drink three or four cups a day. NEVER STEEP HERBS IN ALUMINUM.

SASSAFRAS
(Bark of the Root)

Botanical name: Sassafras officinale. Common name: Ague tree, saxifrax, cinnamon wood, saloip. Medicinal properties: Aromatic, stimulant, alterative, diaphoretic, diuretic.

Often called a spring medicine to purify the blood and cleanse the entire system. Good to flavor other herbs which have a disagreeable taste, and much used in combination with other blood-purifying herbs. Useful as a tonic to stomach and bowels. Will relieve gas. Taken warm, is an excellent remedy for spasms. Valuable in colic, and all skin diseases and eruptions. Good wash for inflamed eyes. Good for kidneys, bladder, chest, and throat troubles. Oil of sassafras is excellent for toothache. Good in varicose ulcers. Wash externally and take internally.

SLIPPERY ELM

We all admire the wonderful slippery elm tree. In my childhood we used to go out with a large knife called a drawshave, and shave off the outer rough bark and then cut off the inner bark in big strips, and carry it home for medical use. It contains various properties which are entirely harmless, and of which even small infants can partake to prevent suffering. Slippery elm is excellent for bowel and bladder troubles, lung troubles, diarrhea, stomach and kidney troubles, boils and inflammations, ulcerated stomach, and bronchitis. It should be in every home, and will save those who use it from much suffering and many doctor's bills.

SUMAC

Botanical name: Rhus glabrum. Common names: Scarlet sumac, smooth sumac, dwarf sumac, upland sumac, Pennsylvania sumac, sleek sumac, mountain sumac. Medical properties: Bark and leaves: Tonic, astringent, alterative, antiseptic. Bernes, diuretic, refringerant, emmenagogue, diaphoretic, cephalic.

A remedy valuable in the cure of gonorrhea and syphilis when others have failed in the following: Equal parts sumac berries and bark, white pine bark, and slippery elm. This tea is very cleansing to the system, and is very useful in leucorrhea, scrofula, and for inward sores and wounds. A tea of sumac berries alone is excellent for bowel complaints, diabetes, all kinds of fevers, and for sores and canker in the mouth there is no superior. Use also as a gargle and wash for the mouth.

TANSY
(Whole Herb)

Botanical name: Tanacetum vulgare. Common names: Hindheel, common tansy. Medical properties: Aromatic, tonic, ennenagogue, diaphoretic, vulnerary. Seed: Vermifuge.

An old well-known family remedy used to tone up the system and soothe the bowels. Excellent taken hot in colds, fevers, la grippe, and agues.

Good for dyspepsia. One of the best remedies to promote menstruation. Tansy seed will expel worms. Useful in hysterics, jaundice, dropsy, worms, and kidney troubles. Strengthens the weak veins. Hot fomentations wrung out of tansy tea is excellent for swellings, tumors, inflammations, bruises, freckles, sunburn, leucorrhea, sciatica, tooth ache, and inflamed eyes. Good in heart trouble. Will check palpitation of the heart in a very short time.

HOLY THISTLE
(Plant)

Botanical name: Centaura benedicta. Common names: Bitter thistle, blessed cardus, spotted thistle. Medicinal properties: Diaphoretic, emetic, tonic, stimulant, febrifuge.

This plant has very great power in the purification and circulation of the blood. It is very effective for dropsy, strengthens the heart, and is good for the liver, lungs, and kidneys. It is soothing to the brain, strengthens the memory, and clears the system of bad humors, and is effective for insanity. It is a good tonic for girls entering womanhood. It is claimed that the warm tea given to mothers will produce a free supply of milk.

It is such a good blood purifier that by drinking a cup of tea twice a day it will cure chronic headaches. Some have called it "blessed thistle" on account of its excellent qualities. About two ounces of the drive plant simmered in a quart of water for two hours makes a tea satisfactory for most purposes. This tea is best taken at bed time as a preventive of disease and it will cause profuse perspiration. Holy thistle is a plant which has been used for centuries. It is very good combined with any of the dock roots (red dock, yellow dock or burdock).

APPENDIX B

Further Notes on Herb Medicine and Midwifery

A cure for diphtheria given by revelation in Arizona or at least is said to have been so given. It is undoubtedly good but on account of the salt-peter should be swallowed only sparingly. Take two ounces of alum and one ounce of salt-peter, pulverize fine and simmer in a pint of home-made molasses. If the molasses cannot be had, use syrup made of sugar, just thick enough to drink. For a small child weaken it. Have it conse-crated like oil.

Huntington, Oliver B. "History of The Life of Oliver B. Huntington. pp 22-23. Available, Zion's Bookstore, Salt Lake City, Utah.

During an interview in May, 1942, Mrs. Ellen Meeks Hoyt, of Orderville, Utah, told me that, "When the Nephites battled with the Lamanites (Book of Mormon peoples), many of them were wounded and badly in need of some kind of remedy .... Their battles fought as far North as these very hills," she said, "and the warriors were cured with the same herbs that grow around us today. Thistle is for our courage; sage is to offset poison. If the soldiers would eat thistle today, they would never be afraid to go into battle."

—Claire Noall

Noall, Claire. "Guardians of the Hearth;" Bountiful, Utah, 1974; p. 16.

Noall, Claire. "Superstitions, Customs, and Prescriptions of Mormon Midwives." California Folklore Quarterly V, In, no. 2, April 1944, P. 109.

The role played by women in the years preceding the era of modern medicine has probably never been adequately recognized. When D. C. Budge began his practice in Logan, almost every town in Cache Valley had one or two practicing midwives. It has been a common thing for writers on medical progress to ridicule these women, who, it must be confessed, were none too well trained in the technical details of delivering and caring for babies.

What they lacked in technical skill, however, they more than made up in common sense, and in a vast sympathy which made them seem like angels of mercy and understanding to the women they attended. Many a grandmother now living looks back with tender appreciation to the momory of some gentle, motherly soul who soothed the fears of her first confinement and later introduced her to the mysteries of caring for her first baby.

Dr. Budge remembers these local midwives of Cache Valley with special appreciation. On the first case he attended he was assisted by Grandma McAllister, the oldest midwife in the valley.... The doctors of the time often blamed these women for the mishaps attending confinements, but D. C. Budge insists that the medical profession could not have done without them. He had an understanding with them that they should handle normal deliveries, feeling free to call on a physician for help in case of trouble. Before the advent of nursing training, they were indispensable to him.

Hayward, Ira N. "Dr. David Clarke Budge—A Pioneer of Western Medicine." Salt Lake City, Utah, 1941; pp. 104-105.

APPENDIX C

ADDITIONAL NOTES ON A PROPER DIET

Anyone familiar with the local supermarket today, will find that most of the big-chain stores carry a wide variety of what is more correctly termed "natural" or "healthy foods." Most have a special section in each one of their individual outlets which handles this sort of menchandise, for those more particularly inclined to the same. Generally higher-priced than the ordinary "refined" foods of the softer line, they offer the shopper his or her choice between the "canned" and "the natural."

Within the past several years, has this new innovation in marketing been added, because of the increased demand by a number of sensible shoppers, ever aware of the growing amount of chemicalization in the present systems of food. Thus, to garner the trade of these particular buyers away from the traditionally-established "health food stores," have the chains introduced this new line of food items within their stores of late.

Also—the national trend toward advertising food products "the more natural way," has become increasingly apparent. Familiar commercials, such as the one in which writer-author Ewell Gibbons extols the virtues of a certain kind of well-known breakfast product, as "my back-to-nature cereal," is indication enough that the trend toward these things is more wide-spread than the average person is now aware of. Other companies have come forth with a multitude of similar products such as "Heartland," "Granola," and a host of others as well.

BIBLIOGRAPHY

Published Works

Anderson, Nels, *Deseret Saints*—The Mormon Frontier in Utah; Chicago, 1942.

Bancroft, Hubert Howe, *History of Utah*; Salt Lake City, 1964.

Book of Mormon.

Caswall, Henry, *The City of The Mormons or Three Days at Nauvoo in 1842*; London, 1842.

Documentary History of The Church in seven volumes; Salt Lake City, 1974.

Guthrie, Douglas, *A History of Medicine*; 1946.

Johnson, Benjamin F., *My Life's Review*; Independence, Missouri, 1947.

Journal of Discourses

Kloss, Jethro, *Back To Eden*; Tennessee, 1939.

Lambert, George C., *Precious Memories* (Sixteenth Book of the Faith-Promoting Series); Salt Lake City, 1914.

Lundwall, Nels B., *Faith Like the Ancients*; Salt Lake City, 1950.

Massengill, Samuel Evans, *Sketch of Medicine and Pharmacy*; Bristol, Tennessee, 1943.

McCoy, Frank, *The Best Way To Health*; Los Angeles, 1926.

Noah, Claire, *Intimate Disciple*; University of Utah Press, 1957.

Richards, Ralph T., *Of Medioine, Hospitals and Doctors*; Salt Lake City, 1953.

Robinson, Phil, *Sinners and Saints*; Boston, 1883.

Rossiter, Frederick M., M.D., *The Practical Guide to Health*; California, 1913.

Smith's Bible Dictionary; Philadelphia, 1948.

Smith, Joseph, *Inspired Version* of the Bible.

Smith, Joseph Fielding, *Teachings of the Prophet Joseph Smith*; Salt Lake City, 1940.

Smith, Lucy, *Joseph Smith and His Progenitors*.

Songs of Zion; Chicago, 1908.

Stokes, Jeremiah, *Modern Miracles*.

Struick, Dirk J., *Yankee Science in the Making*; Boston, 1948.

Tyler, Daniel W., *A Concise History of the Mormon Battalion in the Mexican War* (1848–1847); Salt Lake City, 1881.

Webseter's New International Dictionary of the English Language; Massachusetts, 1946.

West, Franklin L., *Life of Franklin D. Richards*; 1924.

Young, John R., *Memoirs of John R. Young*; Salt Lake City, 1920.

Allen, James B. and Richard O. Cowan, *Mormonism in the Twentieth Century,* BYU, Provo, 1969.

Annals of Medical History, June 1925.

Bulletin of the Medical Library Association, January 1936.

California Folklore Quarterly, April 1944.

California Historical Quarterly, April 1944.

Carter, Kate B., *Pioneer Midwives*; DUP Lesson for April, 1963.

Carter, Kate B., *Pioneer Woman Doctors*; DUP Lesson for March, 1963.

Deseret News, October 24, 1855.

Deseret Weekly News, Volume 49.

Hodapp, Minnie I., *Book of Remembrance* (The Christian Olsen Family); Provo, 1950.

Improvement Era, Volume 42.

Juvenile Instructor, Volume 35.

Lee, Hector, *The Three Nephites*; Albuquerque, New Mexico, 1949.

Long, J. V., *Report of The First General Festival of The Renowned Mormon Battalion*; St. Louis, 1855.

New York Spectator, Tuesday, September 21, 1831.

Relief Society Bulletin, Volume One.

Sessions, Gene A., *Mormon Democrat—The Religious and Political Memoirs of James Henry Moyle*; L.D.S. Church Library, Salt Lake City, 1975.

Utah Historical Quarterly, Volume 10; "Journal of Priddly Meeks" and other articles quoted.

Young Woman's Journal, Volume Two.

Archival Material

"A History of George C. Spilsbury," by himself; Special Collections, Harold B. Lee Library, Brigham Young University, Provo, Utah.

"Autobiography of Violet Ure," by herself; Church Historian's Office, Salt Lake City.

"Diary of Emily Dow Partridge Young;" Special Collections, Harold B. Lee Library, Brigham Young University, Provo, Utah.

"Diary of Isaiah Moses Coombs;" typescript copy in author's possession, Manti, Utah.

"Far West Record;" L.D.S. Church Historian's Office, Salt Lake City, Utah.

"History of Martha Mariah Hancock;" typescript copy in possession of the author.

"Journal of Jared Carter;" Church Historian's Office, Salt Lake City.

"Journals of Joseph Smith;" Church Historian's Office, Salt Lake City.

"Journals of Wilford Woodruff;" Church Historian's Office, Salt Lake City.

"Journal History of the Church;" microfilmed account in Church Library, Salt Lake City.

"Minutes of the Female Relief Society of Nauvoo;" Church Historian's Office, Salt Lake City.

Oral Interviews

Mrs.—(Anonymous)—, Orem, Utah; Summer of 1972; conducted by the author.

Mrs. Elvira Dastrup, Richfield, Utah; August 8, 1973; conducted by author's father and brother.

Ann Wallis, Salt Lake City; 1952; conducted by author's father at University of Utah Library.

CEDAR FORT, INCORPORATED
Order Form

Name:_____

Address: _____

City: _____ State: _____ Zip: _____

Phone: (   ) _____ Daytime phone: (   ) _____

Joseph Smith And Herbal Medicine

Quantity: _____ @ $12.95 each: _____

plus $3.49 shipping & handling for the first book: _____

(add 99¢ shipping for each additional book)

Utah residents add 6.25% for state sales tax: _____

TOTAL: _____

Bulk purchasing, shipping and handling quotes available upon request.

Please make check or money order payable to:

Cedar Fort, Incorporated.

Mail this form and payment to:

Cedar Fort, Inc.

925 North Main St.

Springville, UT 84663

You can also order on our website **www.cedarfort.com**

or e-mail us at sales@cedarfort.com or call 1-800-SKYBOOK